PHYSIOTHERAPY OF THE SHOULDER

AF652591

PHYSIOTHERAPY OF THE SHOULDER

PP Mohanty PhD
Associate Professor and Head
Department of Physiotherapy
Swami Vivekanand National Institute of
Rehabilitation Training and Research (SVNIRTAR)
Cuttack, Odisha, India

Monalisa Pattnaik MPT
Assistant Professor, Physiotherapy
Swami Vivekananda National Institute of
Rehabilitation Training and Research
Cuttack, Odisha, India

JAYPEE *The Health Sciences Publishers*
New Delhi | London | Philadelphia | Panama

JAYPEE

Jaypee Brothers Medical Publishers (P) Ltd.

Headquarters

Jaypee Brothers Medical Publishers (P) Ltd
4838/24, Ansari Road, Daryaganj
New Delhi 110 002, India
Phone: +91-11-43574357
Fax: +91-11-43574314
Email: jaypee@jaypeebrothers.com

Overseas Offices

J.P. Medical Ltd
83, Victoria Street, London
SW1H 0HW (UK)
Phone: +44 20 3170 8910
Fax: +44 (0)20 3008 6180
Email: info@jpmedpub.com

Jaypee Medical Inc.
The Bourse
111 South Independence Mall East
Suite 835, Philadelphia, PA 19106, USA
Phone: +1 267-519-9789
Email: jpmed.us@gmail.com

Jaypee Brothers Medical Publishers (P) Ltd
Bhotahity, Kathmandu, Nepal
Phone: +977-9741283608
Email: kathmandu@jaypeebrothers.com

Jaypee-Highlights Medical Publishers Inc
City of Knowledge, Bld. 237, Clayton
Panama City, Panama
Phone: +1 507-301-0496
Fax: +1 507-301-0499
Email: cservice@jphmedical.com

Jaypee Brothers Medical Publishers (P) Ltd
17/1-B Babar Road, Block-B, Shaymali
Mohammadpur, Dhaka-1207
Bangladesh
Mobile: +08801912003485
Email: jaypeedhaka@gmail.com

Website: www.jaypeebrothers.com
Website: www.jaypeedigital.com

© 2015, Jaypee Brothers Medical Publishers

The views and opinions expressed in this book are solely those of the original contributor(s)/author(s) and do not necessarily represent those of editor(s) of the book.

All rights reserved. No part of this publication may be reproduced, stored or transmitted in any form or by any means, electronic, mechanical, photocopying, recording or otherwise, without the prior permission in writing of the publishers.

All brand names and product names used in this book are trade names, service marks, trademarks or registered trademarks of their respective owners. The publisher is not associated with any product or vendor mentioned in this book.

Medical knowledge and practice change constantly. This book is designed to provide accurate, authoritative information about the subject matter in question. However, readers are advised to check the most current information available on procedures included and check information from the manufacturer of each product to be administered, to verify the recommended dose, formula, method and duration of administration, adverse effects and contraindications. It is the responsibility of the practitioner to take all appropriate safety precautions. Neither the publisher nor the author(s)/editor(s) assume any liability for any injury and/or damage to persons or property arising from or related to use of material in this book.

This book is sold on the understanding that the publisher is not engaged in providing professional medical services. If such advice or services are required, the services of a competent medical professional should be sought.

Every effort has been made where necessary to contact holders of copyright to obtain permission to reproduce copyright material. If any have been inadvertently overlooked, the publisher will be pleased to make the necessary arrangements at the first opportunity.

Inquiries for bulk sales may be solicited at: jaypee@jaypeebrothers.com

Physiotherapy of the Shoulder

First Edition: **2015,** Reprint: 2023

ISBN 978-93-5152-569-1

Printed in India

Dedicated to

Baba,

Without your love, we would not have been able to achieve our goal.

Preface

Physiotherapy of the Shoulder is written to meet the needs of the students and clinicians. The first chapter of the book covers the basic anatomy and the biomechanics of the shoulder, knowledge of which is essential to understand the mechanical problems. Evaluation and assessment is the key for appropriate planning of the physiotherapy management of any problem, without which successful management may not be possible. We have tried our best to include as much evidence as possible. Almost all the shoulder problems related to physiotherapy are included, so it will be convenient to get the overall physiotherapy management of the mechanical shoulder problems in one book. We hope this book may provide useful guidance to the students and the clinicians. The authors would like to receive feedback and modification from the readers.

PP Mohanty
Monalisa Pattnaik

Acknowledgments

We would like to thank Dr BM Pradhan, Ex-Director, SVNIRTAR, for his constant encouragement and support.

The following people have been invaluable source of information: Our friends Mr CR Mishra, MPT student; Mr Jince Thomas Matthew; and Mrs Raviputi Aruna, Ex-BPT student.

We would also like to thank the undergraduate and postgraduate students Mr Dilip Birwal, Mr Subhasis Swain, Mr Saderson and Miss Deepa for their help for the photography.

Contents

Chapter

1

Anatomy and Biomechanics

It is a complex joint consisting of glenohumeral, acromio-clavicular, sterno-clavicular, scapulo-thoracic and the articulation between coracoacromial arch and greater tuberosity. Acromioclavicular, sternoclavicular and scapulothoracic joints form a closed kinetic chain, i.e. movement in one joint causes motion in the other.

GLENOHUMERAL JOINT

It is a ball and socket type of synovial joint, formed by the articulation of glenoid cavity of scapula and head of humerus. Glenoid cavity is part of a larger sphere with the angular value of about 75°, whereas head of humerus is almost half of a smaller sphere with angular value about 150° (Fig. 1.1). From geometry it is clear that glenohumeral joint is incongruent. The shallow acetabulum is deepened by glenoid labrum, which is a fibrocatilaginous structure with triangular in cross-section, i.e. thicker at periphery and thinner inwards. It, somehow, compensates the incongruity.

Head of humerus makes an angle of about 45° with the shaft. Glenoid cavity faces upward, forward and outward, whereas head faces upward, backward and inward.

The thin and lax joint capsule is attached to the margin of glenoid labrum proximally and to the neck of humerus distally. It is loosely attached anteroinferiorly and inferiorly forms a

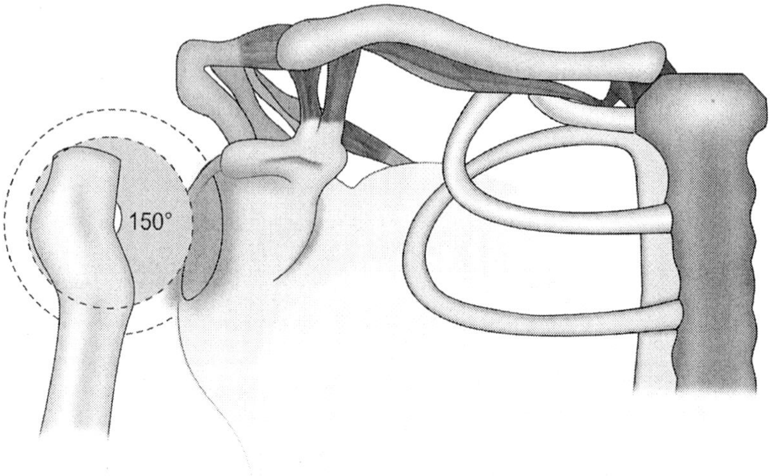

Fig. 1.1: Osseous anatomy of the shoulder girdle

redundant fold which allows a wide range of abduction. The ligaments are so loosely attached that the head can be distracted 2 cm outward with the arm by the side. 55° of abduction, 30° of horizontal flexion is referred as resting position of the shoulder joint, where the joint space and volume are maximum, capsule-ligamentous structures are maximally laxed and joint is least stable. At this position the head of the humerus can be distracted by 3 cm outward. With the arm by the side superior joint capsule remains taut, whereas remainder of the capsule twisted forward and medially. The posterior capsule tightens when the arm rotates internally. External rotation is limited by the anterior joint capsule, middle glenohumeral ligament, anterior band of coracohumeral ligament and subscapularis muscle. The rotator cuff tendons, i.e. supraspinatus, infraspinatus, teres minor and subscapularis blend with the fibers of joint capsule. Stability is sacrificed for mobility due to bony architecture and loosely attached capsule.

The capsule is reinforced by glenohumeral and coracohumeral ligaments. The middle glenohumeral ligament reinforces the capsule anteriorly and checks external rotation, whereas inferior glenohumeral ligament strengthen the capsule anteroinferiorly preventing anterior subluxation and dislocation. The coracohumeral ligament strengthens the superior joint capsule. With the arm by the side the stability of the joint is maintained by both superior joint capsule and coracohumeral ligament, provided the glenoid cavity is oriented normally, i.e. faces upward and outward. The anterior band of coracohumeral ligament checks external rotation and extension, whereas the posterior band checks internal rotation and flexion. The transverse humeral ligament traverses the bicipital groove preventing displacement of long head of biceps.

ACROMIOCLAVICULAR JOINT

Clavicle is a S-shaped bone, the lateral third being concave anteriorly and horizontally placed. The convex articulating surface of clavicle articulates with the plane/concave articulating surface of acromion process, which faces anteromedially. Acromioclavicular joint is less mobile as it is a plane synovial joint.

It has a weak thin capsular ligament which is reinforced by strong superior and inferior acromioclavicular ligaments and coracoclavicular ligaments. Superior and inferior acromioclavicular ligaments prevent over-riding of clavicle on the acromion.

Coracoclavicular ligament is very important in providing acromioclavicular joint stability. It has got two parts—horizontally oriented trapezoid ligament and vertically oriented conoid ligament. The horizontally oriented trapezoid ligament checks over-riding or lateral movement of clavicle on the acromion. It also checks excessive narrowing of scapuloclavicular angle as viewed from above. The vertically oriented conoid ligament checks superior movement of clavicle on the acromion. It also checks excessive widening of scapuloclavicular angle as viewed from above. As the arm abducts, scapula rotates outward increasing the distance between the clavicle and coracoid process, pulling the conoid ligament taut. The tension of the conoid ligament rotates the clavicle backward resulting into elevation of lateral end of clavicle.

STERNOCLAVICULAR JOINT

Convex clavicular surface articulates with sternum and the 1st rib. Medial end of clavicle is concave anteroposteriorly and convex vertically, articulates with the curved notch of manubrium of the sternum. It is a saddle-shaped synovial joint, so freely movable in almost all planes.

It has capsular ligament which is reinforced by anterior and posterior sternoclavicular ligament, superiorly by interclavicular ligament, costoclavicular ligament and intra-articular disc. Intra-articular disc separates joint cavity into 2 compartments and checks medial displacement of clavicle. Costoclavicular and sternoclavicular ligaments strongly anchor the medial end of clavicle to the sternum. The short and strong costoclavicular ligament provide stability to SC joint during clavicular rotation associated with shoulder elevation. The anterior band of costoclavicular ligament is directed upward and laterally to check excessive upward rotation of clavicle, whereas the posterior band of costoclavicular ligament is directed upward and medially to check excessive downward rotation of clavicle.

Scapulothoracic joint is not a true anatomical joint because it has no usual joint characteristics. It is a functional joint. The superior angle of scapula lies level with T2 spinous process, root of spine of scapula lies level with T3 spinous process and inferior angle of scapula lies level with T7spinous process. Scapula makes an angle of about 30° in the frontal plane and scapuloclavicular angle is about 60°as viewed from above with arm by the side. The vertebral border of scapula is parallel to the spine and positioned approximately 3 inches from the midline of the thorax.

Suprahumeral joint is an articulation between the head of humerus and coracoacromial arch. Coracoacromial arch forms an important protective arch over the glenohumeral joint to prevent superior dislocation of head of humerus and protect the glenohumeral joint from direct overhead trauma. It is the potential site for impingement of suprahumeral structures like supraspinatus, infraspinatus, long head of biceps and subacromial bursa.

Bursae

Bursa is a closed cavity, lined by synovium, present between two anatomical structures to prevent friction during movements. There are about 8–9 bursae around the shoulder joint, out of which only 2 are important clinically.

Subacromial/subdeltoid bursa lies over the supraspinatus tendon underneath the acromion and deltoid muscle. It usually does not communicate with the joint cavity. Rupture of calcific supraspinatus tendonitis communicate it with the joint cavity giving rise to secondary bursitis. Inflammed bursa is susceptible to impingement underneath the coracoacromial arch.

Subscapularis bursa lies over the anterior joint capsule underneath the subscapularis. It communicates with the joint cavity. So joint effusion manifests clinically by anterior swelling.

Nerve Supply

The spinal roots supplying the rotator cuff and the articular structures are C5, 6, 7. Ligaments, capsule and synovium are supplied by axillary, suprascapular, subscapular, thoracoacromial and musculocutaneous nerves. Axillary artery, circumflex humeral arteries supply to the shoulder joint and axillary vein is the main vein.

Blood Supply of the Rotator Cuff Tendons

The rotator cuff tendons include supraspinatus, infraspinatus, teres minor and subscapularis which blend with the fibers of joint capsule to form a continuous cuff surrounding the posterior, superior and anterior aspects of the humeral head. It provides dynamic stabilization for the joint.

The blood supply to the rotator cuff is derived from 6 vessels. Anterior humeral circumflex, the bony branch supplying supraspinatus and postcircumflex humeral and suprascapular arteries supplying infraspinatus and teres minor are always present. Thoracoacromial artery supplying supraspinatus is sometimes absent. Suprahumeral and subscapular arteries are often absent. The suprascapular and subscapular arteries are muscular branches. In the dependent arm the arteries are elongated and compressed, compromising the circulation. During arm elevation, abduction and flexion contraction of rotator cuff compresses the arteries producing ischemia. The area within the conjoint rotator cuff tendons is relatively avascular and develops ischemia, is referred as critical zone. Blood supply to supraspinatus and to a lesser extent the infraspinatus are relatively poor. Supraspinatus and infraspinatus to a lesser extent are frequently degenerated due to nutritional deficit either with normal level of activities or from increased level of activities. The incidence tends to increase with advancing age.

BIOMECHANICS

In normal standing posture the antecubital fossa faces anteriorly and the olecranon faces posteriorly with the palm of the hand facing the body. The proximal and distal ends of the humerus should be in the same vertical plane when viewed from side, front or back.

Stability

In normal standing with the arm by the side, the tension of superior joint capsule and coracohumeral ligament are responsible for the stability of the shoulder joint, provided the glenoid cavity faces upward and outward. So minimal rotator cuff muscle activity is required to support the weight of the hanging arm. Once the arm elevates from the side, the tension of superior joint capsule and coracohumeral ligament is lost, so rotator cuff muscles must act to hold the head of humerus within the glenoid cavity during movement of the arm.

With head forward posture there is increased upper cervical lordosis, increased cervicothoracic kyphosis, rounded shoulders with depression and protraction of scapulae and reduced scapuloclavicular angle (thoracic outlet). With the loss of normal scapular orientation the tension of superior joint capsule is lost, so rotator cuff muscles must act to provide stabilization of glenohumeral joint, even while the arm is by the side. Overactivity of rotator cuff muscles at rest to compensate for capsular stabilization results in increased tensile stress to the joint capsule, with which it blends. There is increased collagen proliferation leading to progressive capsular fibrosis and thickening. Loss of extensibility of joint capsule predisposes to periarthritis.

In flaccid hemiplegia, flaccid paralysis of the scapular muscles, changes the normal orientation of the glenoid cavity. In upright position there is loss of tension of superior joint capsule, which normally demands compensatory activity of rotator cuff muscles. But flaccid paralysis of rotator cuff fails to act to support the weight of the hanging arm, giving rise to inferior subluxation/dislocation of humeral head.

With the arm by the side, the joint capsule is twisted forward and medially. During arm abduction the capsule is progressively twisted pulling the head of humerus against the glenoid cavity and at a point no further movement is possible, referred as closed pack position. At the closed pack position capsulo-ligamentous structures are taut, space between the head of humerus and the glenoid cavity is the minimum and greater tubercle comes in contact with coracoacromial arch. It requires external rotation of arm to allow further movement. With external rotation, twisted and taut capsule becomes untwisted and lax, greater tubercle clears the coracoacromial arch allowing further abduction. Forceful abduction in the absence of external rotation impinges the greater tubercle against the coracoacromial arch. Therefore, in case of periarthritis one must restore external rotation before mobilizing for shoulder abduction.

Movements

Normally during initial shoulder abduction up to about 30°, there is pure glenohumeral abduction during which scapular muscles act statically to fix the scapula and prepare for subsequent dynamic action. The downward and inward pull of rotator cuff and upward and outward pull of deltoid form a force couple about the axis of glenohumeral joint (Fig. 1.2), which abducts the joint. Beyond 30° of abduction scapula begins to move and there is glenohumeral and scapulothoracic joints motion with 2:1 ratio. For every 15° abduction-elevation, there is 10°glenohumeral abduction and 5° scapulothoracic elevation. Much of the scapular movement occurs because of movement at sternoclavicular joint; the clavicle protracts about 30°, elevates about 30° and rotates about 50°. Acromioclavicular joint contributes less because its planar surfaces do not allow much angular movement. Upper and lower trapezius and serratus anterior muscles form another force couple moving the scapula forward on the rib cage and rotates upward about the axis of acromioclavicular joint, while levator scapulae and rhomboids balance the unwanted action of above muscles. Scapular movement contributes about 30° of arm elevation. The scapuloclavicular angle, as viewed from above, reduces

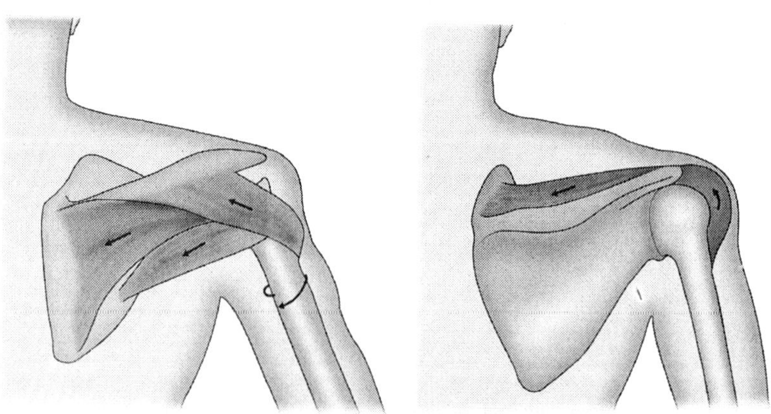

Fig. 1.2: Rotator cuff and deltoid force couple

from 60° to 50°. With the scapular rotation, tightening of the conoid ligament pulls the clavicle into backward rotation resulting into elevation of lateral end of clavicle, which combined with acromioclavicular joint movement contributes about 30° of arm elevation. Combined glenohumeral and scapular movements produce about 160° of arm elevation, about 100° at glenohumeral and about 60°scapular joints. Remaining movement occurs as a result of spinal bending away from the side of arm movement. If both the arms elevate simultaneously the cervicothoracic spine extends backward to allow further elevation.

Teres minor and infraspinatus act as lateral rotators to clear greater tuberosity from the undersuface of coraco-acromial arch. The long head of biceps, which originates from the superior lip of glenoid fossa is intracapsular but extra-synovial. It helps in shoulder abduction when arm is externally rotated. The downward glide of humeral head has been attributed to bicep tendon, infraspinatus and teres minor, which is essential for prevention of impingement of suprahumeral structures against the coracoacromial arch.

ARTHROKINEMATICS OF SHOULDER MOVEMENTS

External Rotation

STJ: Scapula adducts as arm retracts

SCJ: Clavicle rotates about long axis

GHJ: The humeral head glides anteriorly

Abduction

STJ: Initial 30°—scapula is set against thorax, 30° to full abduction; the scapula rotates upwardly and forward around rib cage.

ACJ: Clavicle glides inferiorly and anteriorly.

SCJ: Clavicle glides inferiorly from 90° to 120°; then clavicle rotates backward along its long axis.

GHJ: The humeral head glides inferiorly and rolls superiorly on the glenoid

Internal rotation

STJ: Scapula abducts as arm protracts

SCJ: Clavicle rotates about long axis

GHJ: The humeral head glides posteriorly

Flexion

STJ: Scapula abducts and upwardly rotates in rhythm with GH movement to maintain muscle length-tension relationship.

ACJ: Clavicle glides superiorly

SCJ: Clavicle glides inferiorly and laterally rotates

GHJ: The humeral head glides inferiorly and posteriorly on the glenoid. Humerus undergoes lateral distraction while spinning internally.

Extension

STJ: Scapula adducts and downwardly rotates
ACJ: Clavicle glides inferiorly and anteriorly
SCJ: Clavicle glides superiorly and medially rotates
GHJ: The humeral head glides superiorly and anteriorly on the glenoid.

Horizontal Abduction (Extension)

STJ: Scapula adducts
ACJ: Distraction
SCJ: Clavicle glides posteriorly
GHJ: The humeral head glides anteriorly

Horizontal Adduction (Flexion)

STJ: Scapula abducts
ACJ: Compression

SCJ: Clavicle glides anteriorly

GHJ: The humeral head glides posteriorly

In case of paralysis/rupture of supraspinatus, deltoid can initiate and abduct the arm up to 90°. The force of deltoid rapidly reduces as it approaches 90°, so it can barely hold the arm against gravity. In case of deltoid paralysis, rotator cuff can produce abduction of arm with 50% of normal force. Excessive superior gliding of humerus by the unopposed pull of deltoid, inadequate inferior gliding by insufficient rotator cuff pull or absence of external rotation during arm abduction and flexion may result in impingement of supraspinatus against coracoacromial arch.

Any object falling on shoulder or when the patient falls on the tip of shoulder, the caudal force drives the acromion down. The clavicle remains stable by the trapezius and sterno-cleidomastoid muscles. Ligamentous sprain results if the force of injury exceeds its inherent strength. The first ligament to be damaged is the trapeziod ligament affecting the aneroposterior stability. Excessive force may damage the conoid ligament affecting the vertical stability. The clavicle is pulled upward by the action of trapezius and sternocleidomastoid muscles and acromion is pulled downward by weight of the arm giving rise to positive step sign. Shoulder movement beyond 90° causes pain due to stress from clavicular rotation.

BIBLIOGRAPHY

1. Bachtol CO: Biomechanics of the shoulder. Clin orthop 1980;146:37-41.
2. Basmajian JV: Factors preventing downward dislocation of the abducted shoulder joint. J Bone Joint Surgery 41 (A): 1959;1182-6.
3. Basmajian JV: Weight bearing by ligaments and muscles. Can J Surg 1961;4:166-70.
4. Grant JCB: Method of anatomy. Edn 7. Baltimore, Williams and Wilkins 1965.
5. Inman VT, Saunders JB, Abbott LC: Observations of the function of the shoulder joint. J Bone Joint Surg 1944;26(A):1-30.
6. Johnston TB: The movements of the shoulder joint: Plea for the use of the 'plane of the scapula' as plane of reference for

movements occurring at the humero-scapular joint. J Bone Joint Surg 1937;25(B):252-60.
7. Joint structure and function - A comprehensive Analysis, Norkins.
8. Kapandji IA: The Physiology of the Joints, Vol 1: Upper Limb. New York, Churchill Livingstone, 1970.
9. Kapanji IA. The physiology of the joint, 5th edn. Churchil livingstone. Vol. 1.
10. Kent BE: Functional anatomy of the shoulder complex: A review. Phys Ther 1971;51:867-88.
11. Laurak Smith. Clinical Kinesiology by Brunn storms, 5th edn.
12. Lockhart RD: Movements of the normal shoulder joint. J Anat 1936;64:288-302.
13. Lucas DB: Biomechanics of the shoulder joint. Arch Surg 1973;107:425-32.
14. MacConaill MH, basmajian JV: Muscles and movements: A Basis for Human Kinesiology. Baltimore, Williams and Wilkins, 1969.
15. Matsen FA: Biomechanics of the shoulder. In: Frankel VH, Nordin M (ed): Basic Biomechanics of the Skeletal System. Philadelphia. Lea and Febiger, 1970.
16. Moore KL: Clinical oriented anatomy 2nd edn. Baltimore, 1985, Williams and Wilkins.
17. Moore KL: Clinically Oriented anatomy. Baltimore, Williams and Wilkins, 1980.
18. Neuman DA. Kinesiology of the musculoskeletal system. 1st edn, Mosby 2002.
19. Peat M: Functional anatomy of the shoulder complex. Phys Ther 1986;66:1855-65.
20. Perry J: Anatomy and biomechanics of the shoulder in throwing, swimming, gymnastics and tennis. Clin Sports Med 1983;2:247-70.
21. Rothman RH, Marvel JP, Heppenstall RB: Anatomical considerations in the glenohumeral joint. Orthop Clin North Am 6 1975;(2):341-52.
22. Sarrafian SK: Gross and functional anatomy of the shoulder. Clin Orthop 1983;173:11-8.
23. Warwick R, Williams P (Eds): Gray's Anatomy, 35th British edn. Philadelphia, WB Saunders, 1973.

Chapter

2

Evaluation of Shoulder Joint

Shoulder and arm is the common site for referred pain from heart, diaphragm, myofascial pain syndrome of the shoulder girdle muscles and radiating pain from the cervical spine. A detailed history followed by screening the suspected joints is essential to rule out involvement of other joints and focus on the shoulder joint having primary pathology.

Screening the Cervical Spine

Before examining the shoulder joint, pathology of the cervical spine should be excluded. A scan examination consists of active movements of cervical spine followed by passive terminal overpressure to elicit the original symptoms. Full and pain free range of motions with passive terminal over pressure exclude the involvement of cervical spine.

HISTORY

a. Site of pain: Pain from shoulder pathology often referred to lateral brachial region (C5 dermatome) and never localized to shoulder joint except acromioclavicular dysfunctions and never goes below the elbow.
b. Patient may find difficulty to lie on affected side shoulder.
c. Activities of daily living
   - Difficulty/ Inability in reaching into the back pocket and fastening bra behind indicates impairment of internal rotation.

- Eating, putting on or removing shirt or banyan, reaching above the shoulder level indicates impairment of abduction and external rotation.

d. Nature of pain
Usually pain experienced during active movement and relieved by rest except subacromial bursitis, where one gets rest pain.

e. Onset of pain
Usually insidious as in tendonitis and capsular tightness, whereas acute bursitis or tendonitis due to trauma are of sudden onset.

f. General health to find out any cardiac, respiratory, gall-bladder or pancreatic diseases.

PHYSICAL EXAMINATION

Observation

a. *Attitude:* Arm may be by the side or held across the chest or supported by other hand. Shoulder may be raised due to muscles spasm. Normally, level of dominant shoulder is lower because of overuse there is over-strengthening and overstretching of scapular muscles.

b. *Function:* Check arm swing during walking, dressing, and general willingness to use arm, etc.

Inspection

a. Skin in relaxed standing position
   - *Color:* red, pale, cyanosed
   - *Texture:* rough, smooth
   - *Moisture:* dry, wet
   - *Scar/blemishes:* present/absent

   Skin could be red, shiny, smooth and moistened suggestive of hypervascularity due to underlying inflammation or increased sympathetic activity.

   Skin could be pale, dry, rough and scaly suggestive of hypovascularity due to chronic inflammation or reduced sympathetic activity.

b. Soft tissues with the patient sitting on a stool and foot flat on ground:
   - Atrophy of scapular and shoulder muscles
   - *Swelling:* Anterior joint swelling implies subscapular bursitis and/or shoulder joint effusion
   - Lateral swelling indicates subdeltoid bursitis
   - Entire arm swelling indicates reflex sympathetic osteodystrophy or immobilization following injury or surgery.

c. *Posture in relaxed standing position:* Check shoulder heights, position of head on neck and neck on trunk

d. *Bony prominences in relaxed standing position:* Check the relationship of the following bony landmarks with each other and from a reference point, ground in standing or some fixed point on body midline (sternal notch, xiphisternum, symphysis pubis) is taken as reference. SC joint, AC joint, position of scapula and clavicle, greater tubercle, lesser tubercle, acromion, humeral epicondyles, olecranon, etc.
   - Distance between acromion to greater tuberosity for inferior subluxation of glenohumeral joint.
   - Rotatory position of humerus by checking position of humeral epicondyles, greater and lesser tuberosities and orientation cubital fossa.
   - *Step sign:* Clavicle is in higher position by the upward pull of trapezius and sternocleidomastoid muscles and acromion lowered by the downward pull of weight of the arm suggestive AC joint subluxation due to sprain coracoclavicular ligament.
   - *Flattening of shoulder:* Normally shoulder contour is rounded. Flattening occurs in dislocation (Anterior dislocation common).

Movements

I. (a) Active Bilaterally Symmetrical Movements in Sitting

Patient sitting erect on a stool and physiotherapist observes standing on the back

Ask the patient to abduct the arm to 90° then elbow flexion to 90°, horizontally extend shoulder and externally rotate the shoulder.

Check from the back for:

- Bilateral synchronous glenohumeral rhythm, disturbed rhythm indicates glenohumeral stiffness, weakness of shoulder muscles or inhibition due to pain.
- Horizontal extension restricted when anterior joint capsule is tight.
- External rotation restricted when anterior joint capsule is tight.
- Oscillatory movements of scapula implies inability to fix due to weakness of scapular muscles or fatigue.

I. (b) Active Movements in Sitting

Scapular elevation, depression, protraction and retraction shoulder flexion, extension, external rotation, internal rotation and abduction.

Check:

- Willingness for the movement indicates severity of the lesion. Patient's unwillingness to do the movement indicates more severe lesion. So one should be careful while examining further.
- *Pain*: Site, the range at which pain starts (P1) and the change in intensity with movement and the range at which pain stops (P2) the movement further. Pain during midrange of abduction implies impingement/painful arc syndrome.
- ROM
- *Quality of movement:* Glenohumeral rhythm and smoothness of movement
- Crepitus: Characteristics of degeneration

II. Passive Glenohumeral Movements with the Scapula Fixed in Lying

Physiotherapist fixes the scapula by one hand and gives passive physiological movements by the other hand. Check and record the following:

- ROM by goniometer
- *End feel:* It is the nature of feel experienced by the examiner at the end of range of motion.

Physiological End Feel

Soft tissue approximation: The muscle bulks come in contact with each other limiting further movement, which can be seen also.

Elastic end feel: Resistance felt is lesser, yields more with passive over pressure, recoils back as the force is released. It is the characteristic of muscle tension.

Leathery: Resistance felt is more, yields less with application of more pressure. It is the characteristic of tension of capsule.

Bony end feel: Whatever amount of terminal over pressure you apply, it does not yield at all. It is the characteristic of bony block.

Pathological End Feel

Empty end feel: No resistance is being felt, but the movement is stopped. It is the characteristic of bursitis.

Springy rebound: It yields with passive over pressure, but recoils back like a spring as the force is released. It is the characteristic of internal derangement.

Muscle spasm end feel: Spasm is associated with pain and elastic end feel.

- Pain: Site, the range at which pain starts and the change in intensity with movement
- Painful arc
- Crepitus.

III. Joint Play in Lying

Check the amplitude of the following joint play movements and pain. Compare it with the sound side and record.

- Posterior glide (AP) of head of humerus over the glenoid fossa – Internal rotation and flexion.
- Anterior glide (PA) of head of humerus over the glenoid fossa – External rotation and extension.

- Inferior glide of head of humerus over the glenoid fossa – For abduction
- Lateral distraction of head of humerus

  Non-contractile tissue (capsule-ligamentous) dysfunction is characterized by abnormal response to passive movement and joint play.
- Reduced amplitude without pain – ankylosed
- Reduced amplitude with pain – adhesion, spasm due to sprain
- Normal amplitude without pain – normal
- Increased amplitude with pain – G II sprain
- Increased amplitude without pain – Rupture of ligament, flaccid paralysis

IV. Resisted Isometric Contraction in Supine

Check strength and pain
- Strong and pain – GI strain
- Strong and no pain – normal
- Weak and pain – G II strain
- Weak and no pain – Complete rupture, paralysis

Contractile tissue (musculotendinous unit) dysfunction is characterized by abnormal response to resisted isometric contraction and passive stretching.
- Internal rotation – subscapularis
- External rotation arm by side – Infraspinatus
- External rotation with arm at 75° of abduction – teres minor
- Abduction of arm close to the side – supraspinatus
- Arm flexion with elbow straight – Biceps brachi
- Elbow flexion/supination – Biceps brachi

Neuromuscular Examination

- *Sensation:* Lateral arm- C5, Lateral forearm- C6, Middle finger - C7, Medial forearm- C8, Medial arm- T1.
- *Muscle power:* Deltoid and Biceps - C5, Biceps and wrist extensors - C6, Triceps and wrist flexors - C7, Hand intrinsics - C8 and T1.

- *Reflexes:* Biceps jerk - C5, Brachioradialis jerk - C6, Triceps jerk - C7, Abductor digiti minimi jerk - C8.

Palpation

Skin: Texture - Smooth/Rough
- *Tenderness:* Present/Absent
- *Temperature:* Normal, cold, warmth
- *Moisture:* Dry/Moist
- *Mobility:* Adherent/Mobile

Soft Tissue

- *Swelling:* Anterior joint swelling implies subscapular bursitis and/or shoulder joint effusion
  - Lateral swelling indicates subdeltoid bursitis
  - Entire arm swelling indicates reflex sympathetic osteodystrophy or immobilization following injury or surgery.

Fluctuation test to check joint effusion, press the swelling on one side of the joint, if the impulse of the dispersed fluid is felt on opposite side or the swelling becomes more prominent on the other side, then the test becomes positive indicative of joint effusion.

- Wasting by girth measurement using flexible measure tape. Measure the circumference at a particular level, at a particular distance from a fixed bony landmark and compare the same with the opposite side.
- Tenderness: At local site -
  - Transverse humeral ligament
  - Long head biceps
  - Supraspinatus
  - Infraspinatus
  - Subscapularis
  - Anterior/posterior joint capsule.
  - Mobility
  - Continuity
  - Consistency: tone

Peripheral pulsation: Radial and brachial artery for rate, depth/ volume, rhythm, proximal-distal deficit.

Bony: SC joint, AC joint, coracoid, greater tubercle, lesser tubercle.

Check the relationship with each other and from reference point.

SPECIAL TESTS

Yergason's Test (Fig. 2.1)

Position of patient: Sitting with arm by the side, in elbow flexed to 90° and FA pronated.

Test: Ask the patient to supinate and externally rotate the shoulder against resistance.

Response: Pain indicates bicipital tendinitis

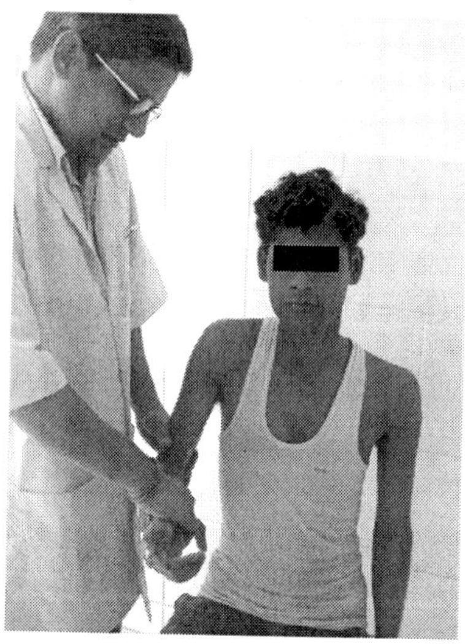

Fig. 2.1: Yergason's test

Speed's Test (Fig. 2.2)

Position of patient: Sitting with arm by the side and elbow straight and forearm supinated.

Test: Resisted shoulder flexion (apply resistance near wrist)

Response: Pain indicates bicipital tendinitis

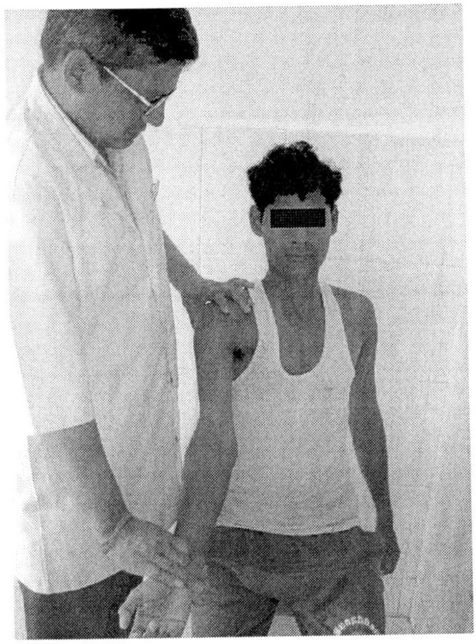

Fig. 2.2: Speed's test

Ludington's Test (Fig. 2.3)

Position of patient: Sitting with clasping both hands behind the head.

Test: Alternate isometric contraction and relaxation of biceps.

Therapist's finger in the bicipital groove, tries to palpate long head of biceps.

Response: Absence of long heads biceps indicates rupture long head of biceps.

Drop Arm Test (Fig. 2.4)

Position of patient: Sitting

Test: Passively take arm up to 90° of abduction and ask the patient to hold it isometrically.

Response: Pain and Inability to hold arm, which falls uncontrollably indicates supraspinatus tear.

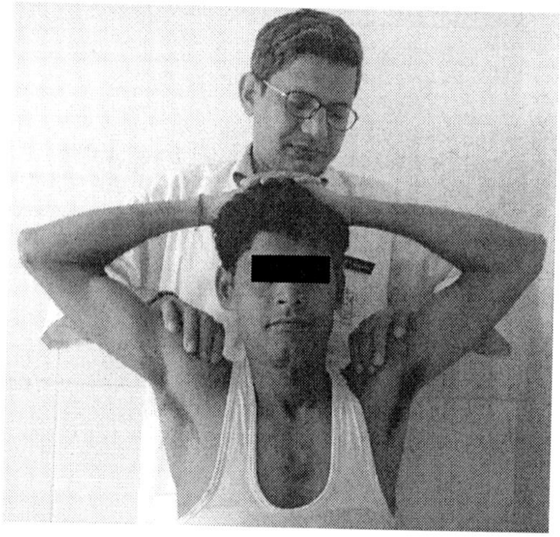

Fig. 2.3: Ludington's test

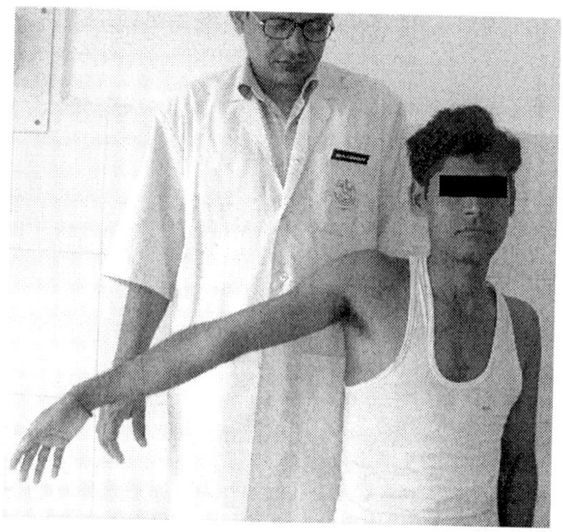

Fig. 2.4: Drop arm test

Empty Can Test/Supraspinatus Test (Fig. 2.5)

Position of patient: Standing with arm horizontally flexion (forward) 30° from 90° abducted position and full internally rotated with thumb facing down.

Test: Resisted abduction.

Response: Pain and weakness indicates supraspinatus tendinitis.

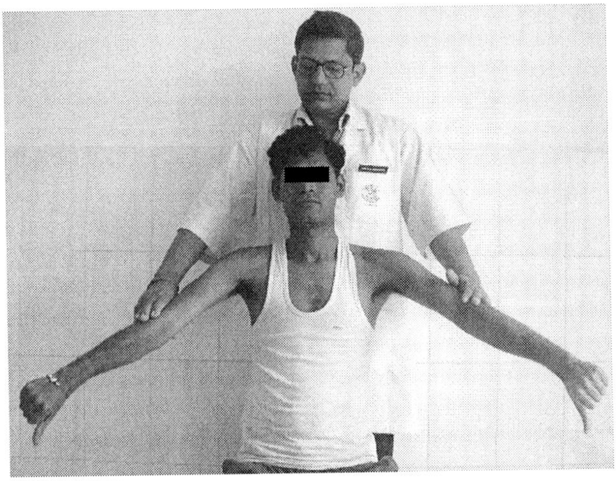

Fig. 2.5: Empty can test

Impingement Sign (Fig. 2.6)

Position of patient: In supine or sitting position, arm by the side and internally rotated.

Test: Passive forward flexion abduction

Response: Painful forward flexion indicates long head of biceps impingement, painful abduction indicates supraspinatus and subdeltoid bursa impingement.

Transverse Humeral Ligament

Position of patient: Sitting

Arm abducted 90°, elbow flexion to 90° and internally rotated. Therapist keeps his finger over bicipital groove.

Test: Ask the patient to externally rotate the shoulder.

Response: Long head of biceps tendon moving out of bicipital groove indicates rupture transverse humeral ligament.

Apprehension Test (Fig. 2.7)

Position of patient: Supine lying/sitting

Therapist standing behind the patient, places one hand over the shoulder with the thumb over the humeral head and other hand grasping the wrist.

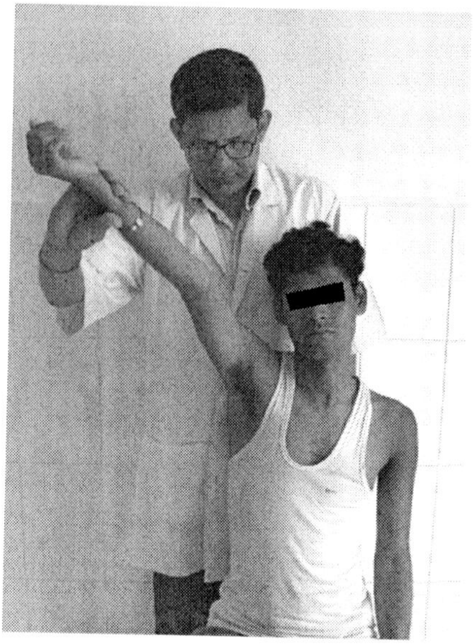

Fig. 2.6: Impingement sign

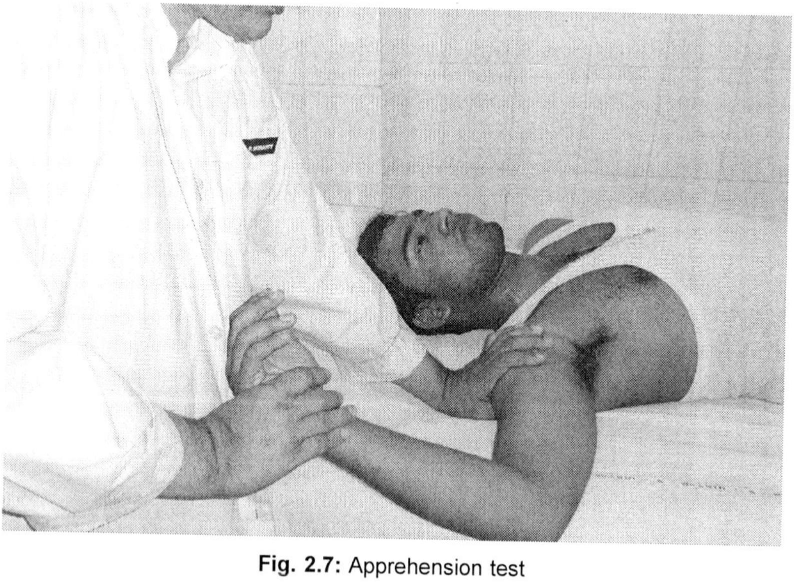

Fig. 2.7: Apprehension test

Test: Arm abducted 90°, elbow flexion to 90° and rotate the shoulder externally by pulling the wrist back, while applying pressure over the back of humeral head forward. Fingers placed on the anterior aspect of shoulder to monitor anterior displacement of head.

Posterior Apprehension Test (Fig. 2.8)

Position of patient: Supine lying/sitting

Therapist standing by the side of the patient places one hand over the shoulder with the thumb over the humeral head and other hand grasping the wrist.

Test: Arm abducted 90°, elbow flexion to 90° and rotate the shoulder internally by pulling the wrist back, while applying pressure over the humeral head pushing it posteriorly.

Allen's Test/Wright's Maneuver (Fig. 2.9)

Position of patient: Sitting

Arm abducted to 90°, horizontally extended, externally rotated and elbow flexed to 90°, turn the head away from the tested side and take a deep breath.

Therapist stands behind and by the side of the patient palpates for the radial pulse.

The test is positive if there is diminution/absence of radial pulse on head rotation and deep inspiration suggestive of thoracic outlet syndrome.

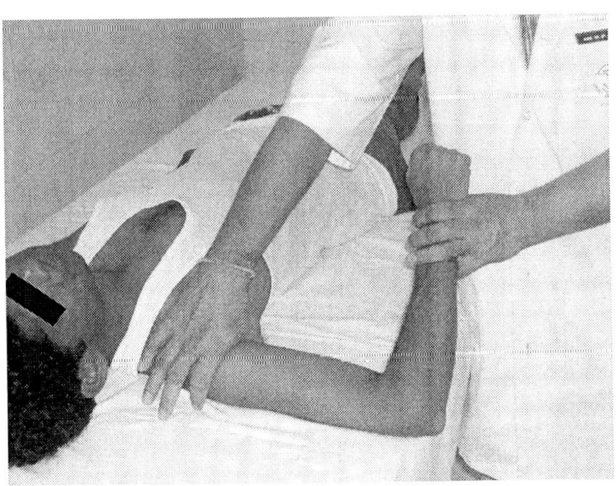

Fig. 2.8: Poterior apprehension test

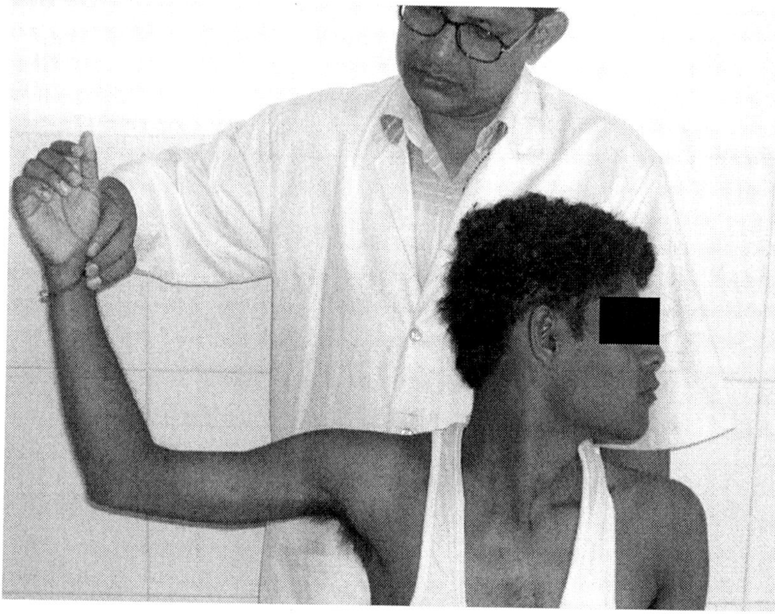

Fig. 2.9: Allen's test

Adson's Test (Fig. 2.10)

Position of patient: Sitting with arm slightly abducted, laterally rotated, hyperextension and retraction.

Therapist stands behind and by the side of the patient palpates for the radial pulse.

Test: Ask the patient to turn head and hyperextend to the tested side, while taking deep breath and hold it for some time.

The test is positive if there is diminution/absence of radial pulse suggestive of TOS due to scalene syndrome.

Costoclavicular Maneuver

Position of patient: Sitting with arm by the side

Therapist stands behind and by the side of the patient palpates for the radial pulse.

Test: Shoulder depression, hyperextension and retraction (exaggerated military posture).

The test is positive if there is diminution/absence of radial pulse suggestive of TOS.

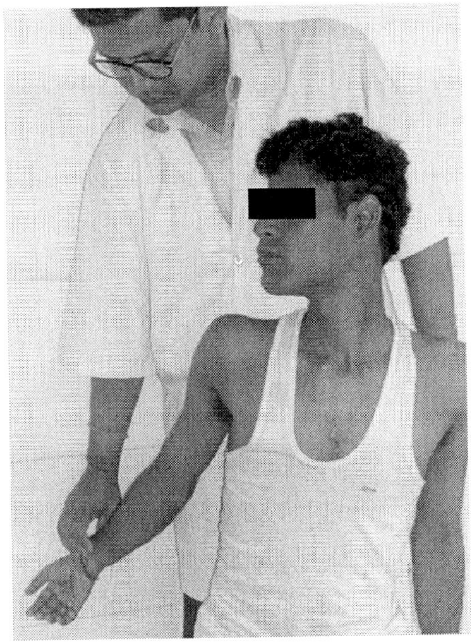

Fig. 2.10: Adson's test

Hyperabduction Test

Position of patient: Sitting with arm by the side

Therapist standing behind the patient palpates for the radial pulse

Test: Hyper abduction of shoulder

The test is positive if there is diminution/absence of radial pulse

Overhead Exercise Test

Position of patient: Sitting with arm elevated.

Test: Rapid flexion and extension of fingers

The test is positive if the symptoms are reproduced or patient complains of asymmetrical heaviness, fatigue, tingling or numbness in the limb. The hand of the affected limb may blanch or discolor when compared with the normal limb.

Elvey's Upper Extremity Tension Test

Position of patient: Supine lying

Test: Abduction of shoulder to 90°, external rotation and extension behind the coronal plane, then elbow extension and forearm supination, then wrist and fingers extension and finally neck side flexion to opposite side is added.

The test is positive if the symptoms are reproduced during either stage of the test indicating median nerve tension test positive.

Similarly tension test for radial nerve can be performed by abduction, internal rotation and extension of shoulder then elbow extension foream pronation and wrist flexion.

Horizontal Adduction Test

Position of patient: Sitting on chair with horizontal adduction of arm.

Therapist standing on back and by the side of patient applies overpressure into horizontal adduction.

Response: Anterior shoulder pain indicates impingement of subscapularis, supraspinatus, long head of biceps, whereas posterior pain indicates infraspinatus, teres minor and posterior capsule.

Superior shoulder pain indicates AC joint pathology.

Paxino's Sign (Fig. 2.11)

Position of patient: Sitting on chair with the arm at the side of chest wall

Therapist standing on back side of patient applies pressure under the acromion towards anterior-superior direction by thumb and counter-pressure inferiorly over clavicle by index finger at the same time.

Response: Pain over AC joint indicates AC joint pathology.

Neer Impingement Test (Fig. 2.12)

Position of patient: Sitting on chair with arm at the side. Therapist standing at side stabilizes scapula by one hand while elevating the internally rotated humerus by another.
Response: Pain and reproduction of symptoms indicates impingement

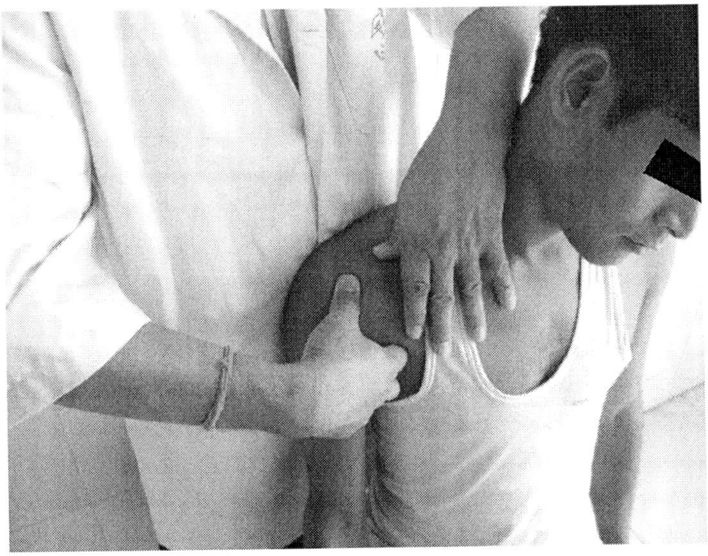

Fig. 2.11: Paxino's test

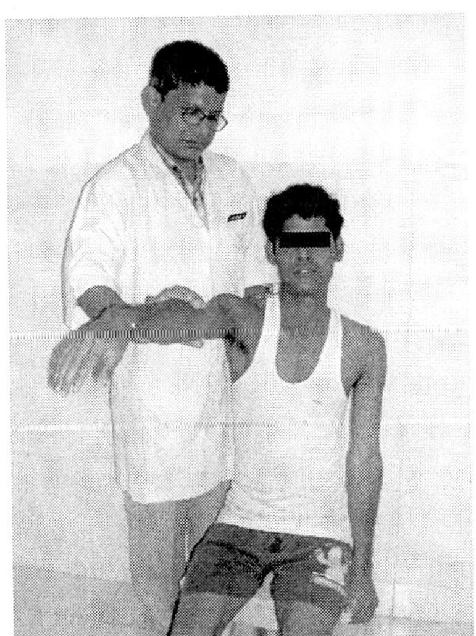

Fig. 2.12: Neer impingement test

Hawkins-Kennedy Impingement Test (Fig. 2.13)

Position of patient: Sitting on the chair with abduction and internal rotation of arm in scapular plane.

Therapist standing at side stabilizes elbow and pushes down on wrist into more internal rotation.

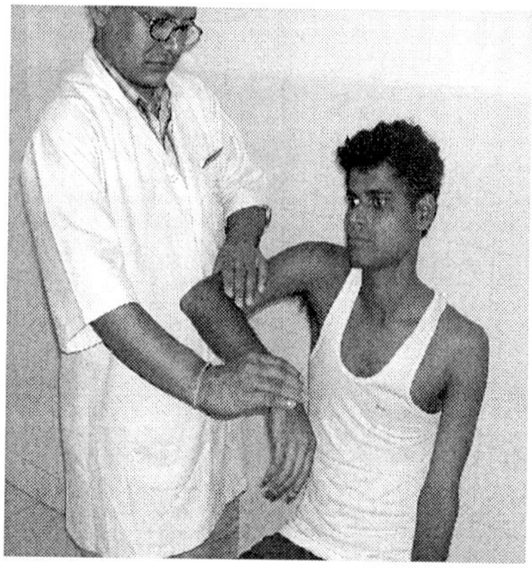

Fig. 2.13: Hawkins-Kennedy impingement test

Response: Pain and reproduction of symptoms indicates impingement.

O' Brien Sign

This test is designed primarily to detect labral tears, but it is also reported to detect the abnormality of acromioclavicular joint. The therapist standing behind the patient asks the patient to forward flex the affected arm 90° with elbow held in full extension. The arm is adducted to 10° to 15° medial to sagittal plane of body and then is internally rotated so that thumb points downward while examiner applies downward force to the arm. With the arm maintained in the same position, this maneuver is repeated with the palm fully supinated. The test is positive if first maneuver causes pain over top of the shoulder or pain is localized to the AC joint and pain is less intense or is absent with second maneuver.

BIBLIOGRAPHY

1. Cyriax J: Textbook of orthopaedic medicine, vol 1: diagosis of soft tissue lesions. Edn 8, London, Bailliere - Tindall 1982.
2. Gould JA III: Orthopaedic and sports physical therapy. Edn 2, St. Louis, Mosby 1990.
3. Hertling D. Kessler RM: Management of common musculoskeletal disorders. Edn 2, Philadelphia, Lippincott 1990.
4. Magee DJ: Orthopaedic physical assessment, Philadelphia, Saunders 1989.

Chapter 3

Impingement Syndrome

The term shoulder impingement syndrome was introduced by Neer (1983) and refers to the compression of rotator cuff, i.e. Supraspinatus, infraspinatus, subacromial bursa and long head of biceps tendon against undersurface of acromion, coracoacromial ligaments and AC joint during arm elevation. This syndrome is characterized by shoulder pain that is exacerbated with arm elevation or overhead activities.

EPIDEMIOLOGY, PREVALENCE AND INCIDENCE

The incidence of shoulder pain in community setting is high, estimated to be 11.2 per 1000 person-years. Chard et al conducted a community survey and found that out of sample of 644 people, 170 (26%) reported shoulder pain with at least 70% subacromial impingement syndrome. A prevalence of 7% has been reported in Swedish population by Jacobson et al. Morrison et al reported in 2000 that 75% of patient presenting with rotator cuff tendonitis had underlying impingement of anterior acromion on the supraspinatus tendon and occasionally infraspinatus. Pink reported shoulder pain in 66% of swimmer, 57% of professional pitcher, 44% of collegiate volleyball player and 20% of collegiate javelin thrower. Several authors have implicated the role of acromioclavicular joint pathology in development of impingement syndrome.

Theory of Impingement

Biomechanical Theory

Initial 30° of abduction takes place in glenohumeral joint.Then movement takes place at glenohumeral and scapulothoracic joints at 2:1 ratio. Elevation of scapula results from the combined movement of SC joint, clavicular rotation and minimal movement at AC joint. At about 60° of abduction there must be external rotation of humerus to move the suprahumeral structures away from the coracoacromial arch in order to avoid impingement. Impairment of shoulder external rotation/scapular motion may result into impingement.

Unbalanced force couple between rotator cuff and deltoid; serratus anterior and trapezeus disturbs the normal shoulder girdle movement and results into impingement syndrome.

Anatomical Theory

The space between greater tubercle and coracoacromial arch is fixed. Reduction of its size due to fracture greater tubercle, AC joint arthritis, etc. or increase in the volume of its content due to edema, fibrosis, calcific deposit, etc. may result in impingement.

Vascular Theory

Main supply to supraspinatus is thoracoacromial artery, which is sometimes absent. Continued over-head activities with the discomfort without rest does not allow it to heal and results into chronic/degenerative tendonitis due to its relative avascularity.

Stages of Impingement Syndrome

Neer described the three classical stages of impingement.

Stage-I involves reversible changes such as edema and hemorrhage of the bursa and cuff is typical in persons under twenty-five years old.

Impingement - Microtrauma - Inflammation/Edema - increased volume of the contents - Further impingement - edema and hemorrhage.

Complaint of toothache like of discomfort following activities, relieved in rest. Impingement sign is positive and painful arc is present.

Stage-II involves irreversible changes such as fibrosis and tendonitis of the rotator cuff, and typically occurs in persons who are twenty-five to forty years old. Collection of inflammatory exudates within its sheath impair circulation, giving rise to gradual degenerative tendonitis, characterized by restriction of movements and crepitus. The tendon substance becomes rough by the lying down of collagen fibers over time giving rise to crepitus. Passive movement is restricted because of fibrous thickening and shortening of the tendon.

Complaint of pain in activities and more in the night. Finds difficulty to lie on affected side shoulder. Resisted isometric contraction of supraspinatus is painful and weak, and passive stretching is restricted and painful.

Stage-III is marked by partial tear or complete tear of rotator cuff and usually is seen in patients over 40 years of age. Attrition of the degenerated tendon over time due to continued overhead activities finally may result into rupture. Rupture is characterized by loss of active movement, while passive movement is present. During abduction there is loss of glenohumeral rhythm; unopposed deltoid action produces more of elevation than abduction.Wasting of supraspinatus, infraspinatus is present and drop arm test is positive.

Later Neer divided impingement into outlet and non-outlet lesions. Outlet impingement occurs when the coracoacromial arch encroaches on the supraspinatus outlet and non-outlet occurs secondarily to thickening or hypertrophy of the bursa or the rotator cuff tendons.

Impingement syndrome can be classified broadly into primary and secondary.

Primary Impingement

Primary mechanical impingement has been described by Neer as impingement of rotator cuff beneath the coracoacromial arch. The cause of impingement process is either by decreasing the subacromial space or by causing a degenerative process of the rotator cuff tendons. It also results from anatomic variation of acromion shape, acromioclavicular joint degenerative arthritis, which is characterized by capsular hypertrophy and spur.

Secondary Impingement

It usually occurs in the younger individual and in athletes and is defined as a relative decrease in supraspinatus outlet caused by instability of the glenohumeral joint. The symptom can be attributed to rotator cuff tendinitis. The symptoms of secondary impingement are often result of rotator cuff overuse as a consequence of multidirectional glenohumeral instability. Scapulothoracic weakness has also been attributed as secondary cause of impingement syndrome due to a lack of scapula stability causing resultant glenohumeral instability. The net effect of secondary causes is usually an anteriosuperior translation of the humeral head, which causes impingement of the cuff against the coracoacromial arch.

Factors contributing to impingement syndrome can be subdivided into intrinsic or extrinsic factors.

FACTORS OF THE INTRINSIC THEORY

Muscle Dysfunction

The primary etiologic factor causing intrinsic changes has been reported to the multiple tension overload of the rotator cuff, especially supraspinatus. When the arm is in the overhead position, eccentric contraction of supraspinatus decelerates internal rotation and adduction of the arm, causing an overload. This phenomenon is most dramatic in sports persons and manual laborers who use overhead motions in their work. This may be caused by the morphology of supraspinatus muscle, which has a greater belly size in comparison to it relatively smaller tendon size. Subsequent fatigue, injury and weakness of the cuff result in instability and muscle imbalance that produce upward humeral migration and subsequent tissue impingement.

Overuse Shoulder

Overuse syndrome also occurs commonly in young competitive athletes and manual laborers who use overhead motion in their work. The inflammation resulting from repetitive micro-trauma increases the area occupied by soft tissues in the subacromial space and leads to friction and wears against coracoacromial arch. The finding of Soslowsky et al described in animal tendons changes that result from over use activity, they are believed to occur in rotator cuff tendons too.

Degenerative Tendinopathy

Uzaki et al studied the pathological changes on the undersurface of the acromion as associated with tears of the rotator cuff in 200 cadaveric shoulders. After radiographic and histological analysis, they found that in the specimens with a partial tear of the cuff, the undersurface of the acromion was almost intact. They concluded that the pathogenesis of most tear is probably a degenerative process. Ogata and Uhthoff suggested that tendon degeneration is the primary etiology of partial tears of the rotator cuff and that they might allow proximal migration of the humeral head, which could result in impingement syndrome.

Relative Ischemia of Rotator Cuff

Intrinsic causes can also be attributed to inflammatory changes within the cuff tendon. These intrinsic factors are related to microvascular pattern of the rotator cuff tendon and to the zone of relative ischemia that occurs in specific arm position as described by Rathburn and Mcnab. This area of relative ischemia is the zone where most pathologic change of the rotator cuff occurs and is known as the critical zone. Its location is approximately 10 mm from insertion of the supraspinatus tendon on the greater tubercle of the humerus. This critical region has therefore been shown to be the area associated with tearing of the supraspinatus tendon.

FACTORS OF THE EXTRINSIC THEORY

Shape of Acromion

Acromial morphology and differences in the shape and slope of the acromion as a potential source of symptoms in the shoulder has been observed. The shape of acromion is classified into type-I (flat), type-II (curved) and type-III (hooked). A higher prevalence of full thickness tears of the rotator cuff was noted in association with type-III acromion. In another study, Morrison evaluated supraspinatus outlet radiographs and found that 80% of eighty-two patients who had tears of the rotator cuff visible in arthrogram had a type-III acromion. Besides acromial morphology age and sex have an independent observation with rotator cuff pathology.

Glenohumeral Instability

Especially in young competitive athletes with symptoms of impingements, it is necessary to consider underlying glenohumeral instability as the primary source of the problem. Glenohumeral subluxation may cause disturbances in the mechanics of overhead motion, which may lead to secondary impingement. This concept may explain why certain throwing athletes do not show improvement after anterior acromioplasty. The underlying instability needs to be treated either with an exercise program designed to strengthen the dynamic stabilizer or with operative intervention if exercise program fails, electromyographic analysis shows that they are all active throughout the act of elevation.

Disturbed Scapulothoracic Rhythm

Sportsmen, typically throwing athletes and swimmers, who suffer from impingement syndrome, have been demonstrated to have dysfunction of the scapulothoracic muscles. The dynamic effect of weakness on the scapular muscles is best seen when the serratus anterior muscle is involved. The inability to protract the scapula gives rise to winging of the scapula when the arm is raised. Weak or unbalanced scapular muscles alter the scapulohumeral rhythm and place a greater strain on glenohumeral articulation, which results in secondary extrinsic impingement.

Os Acromiale

Os acromiale is an unfused distal acromial epiphysis first described by Grube in 1863. Folliasson classified the lesion into four distinct types on the basis of anatomical location, with mesoacromion being the most common type. The prevalence of os acromiale, as reported in both radiographic and anatomical studies, has varied a great deal, with a range of 1 to 15 per cent. It is difficult to detect an os acromiale on a routine anteroposterior radiograph, and an axillary radiograph may thus be needed. An association between os acromiale and impingement syndrome and rotator cuff tears has been reported. Impingement may occur because the unfused epiphysis on the anterior aspect of the acromion may be hypermobile and may tilt anteriorly as a result of its attachment to the coracoacromial ligament. Hertel et al recommended stable fusion of a sizeable and hypermobile os acromiale.

Internal Impingement

Struhn in recent publication introduces the concept of internal impingement. It is due to the contact between the posterior superior glenoid labrum and the posterior aspect of supraspinatus tendon or the superior aspect of the infraspinatus tendon or both at the insertion in the greater tuberosity. It is usually seen with arm use that involves abduction and extreme of external rotation, such as late cocking stage of pitching.

Subcoracoid Impingement

Coracoid impingement is newly examined entity causing anterior shoulder pain that usually occurs with forward flexion and internal rotation. This type of impingement occurs in the coracoid humeral compartment which is the space located between coracoid tuberosity and lesser tubercle of humerus. This space contains subcoracoid bursa, subscapularis bursa and tendon.

The Role of the Acromioclavicular Joint in Impingement Syndrome

Despite its small size, the acromioclavicular joint plays a vital part in upper extremity function; it is necessary in all movement of the arms and scapula. The supraspinatus outlet consists of superior aspect of the humerus, inferior surface of acromion, acromioclavicular joint and roof of the glenohumeral joint namely coracoacromial ligament. The subacromial space contains the tendons of the rotator cuff (supraspinatus, infraspinatus and teres minor), the long head of the biceps and subdeltoid bursa. The height of the space in healthy shoulders is between 9 and 10 mm, whereby with radiographic measurement of less than 6 mm, is pathologic for compression of the rotator cuff. The actual thickness of the rotator cuff tendon in this area is 5 to 6 mm leaving very little clearance in case of enlargement of bursa, hypertrophy of capsule of AC joint and spur, etc.

The rotator cuff contacts the under surface of AC joint with as little as 60° of glenohumeral abduction and in the habitual position of 60° of internal rotation. By 70° degree of abduction, the greater tuberosity of the humerus lies directly beneath AC joint.[15] Biomechanical data has demonstrated the impingement force between two structures to range from 0.42 X body weight in a static cadaveric model to 0.15 X body weight in a dynamic shoulder model. Early degenerative changes at AC joint such as capsular hypertrophy and marginal osteophytes formation may therefore result in cuff irritation.

Clinical Features

Patient complaints of insidious onset of pain over the lateral brachial region (C5, C6). Sharp pain experienced during overhead activities.

Inspection

Atrophy of supraspinatus and infraspinatus muscles.

Movements

Active Abduction → Painful arc present during abduction and elevation.
Passive abduction elevation → Painful arc may be present.
Passive internal rotation → May be painful and restricted
RIC for supraspinatus, infraspinatus or long head of biceps painful and weak.

Palpation

Fibrous thickening and tenderness of suprahumeral structures may be present.

Treatment

- Prevent from further damage by avoiding precipitating overhead activities.
- To resolve inflammation and allow for healing.
- Prevent from recurrence.
- To return back to activities as early as possible.

Ultrasound: Micro massage effect resolves edema and heating effect increases circulation to promote healing.

Cyriax's deep transverse friction massages rearranges proliferated collagen tissues in a functional way, i.e. perpendicular to the direction of stress, one of the most effective manners to withstand the stress. It also disperses inflammatory exudates relieving pain and preventing adhesion. It prevents/breaks the adhesion and increases the extensibility and restores mobility.

For supraspinatus, patient in half-lying position with the hand behind the back (internal rotation) to move its tendon anteriorly out of the undersurface of acromion.

Therapist standing behind and back of the affected side places the index finger reinforced by middle finger over the exact spot and applies to and fro movements across the direction of tendon fibers with adequate pressure and sweep. As the initial pain and discomfort disappears gradually increases the pressure and again as the pain and discomfort disappear gradually increases the pressure further. The frequency of movement is 2/second. The treatment is applied for about 10 minute followed by active movements and passive stretching.

Stretching and mobilization to restore full range of pain free movements reduces pain and prevents recurrence.

To prevent recurrence progressive strengthening of rotator cuff (Fig. 3.1) to balance it with deltoid and balancing scapular rotators, trapezius and serratus anterior force couple is very important.

Townsend, et al examined glenohumeral muscles by EMG analysis during a shoulder rehabilitation program. Result showed that four exercises [Scaption (Fig. 3.2) with internal rotation, horizontal abduction in external rotation, flexion and press-up] were responsible for high level of EMG activity in all muscles. The leading exercise for infraspinatus and teres minor was horizontal abduction with external rotation.

Takeda, et al found that both abduction in the plane of scapula with arm externally rotated and abduction in plane of scapula with the arm in internal rotation (Fig. 3.2) are effective for supraspinatus strengthening. Pushup plus exercises were

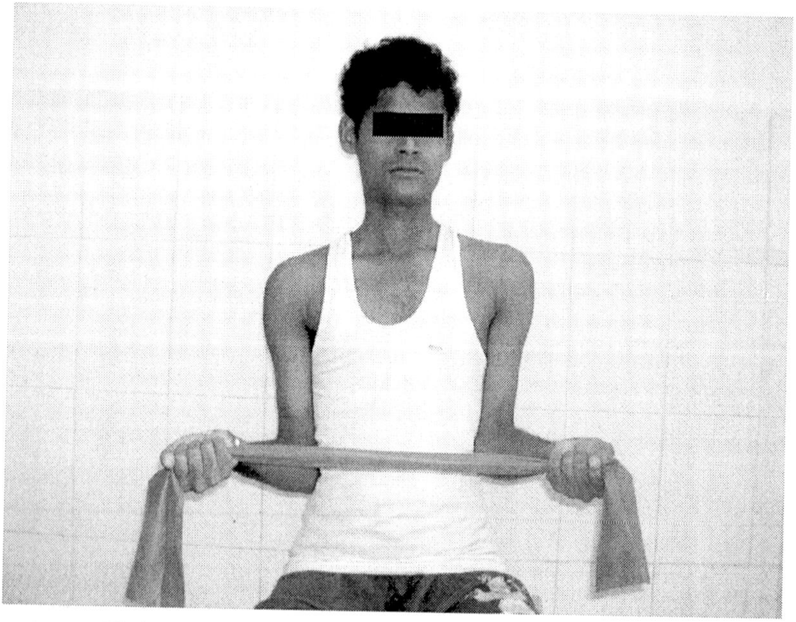

Fig. 3.1: Bilateral resisted external rotation using theraband

superior to internal rotation exercise in activating both parts of subscapularis.

Moseley, et al performed an EMG study of shoulder muscle in nine subjects during sixteen different exercises. He recommended the four core exercises program for scapular muscles. They are scaption, rowing (Fig. 3.3), pushup with a plus and press-up.

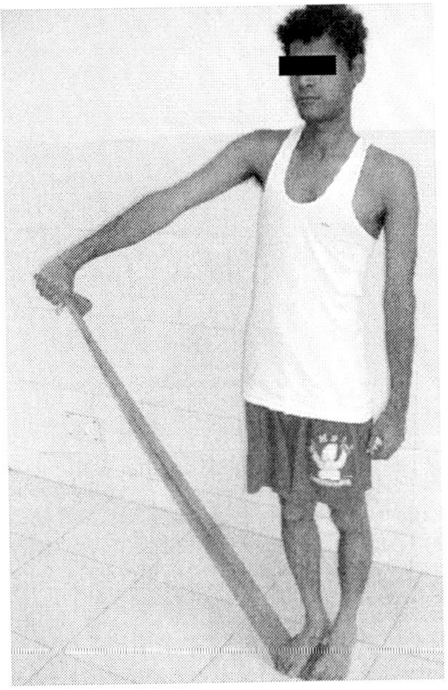

Fig. 3.2: Scaption supraspinatus strengthening in plane of scapula with arm IR

Ekstrom et al analyzed exercises for the trapezius and serratus anterior muscles by surface EMG and demonstrated that the shoulder horizontal extension with external rotation, shoulder shrug exercises, shoulder external rotation at 90° of humeral abduction, a combination of shoulder flexion, horizontal flexion and external rotation best activated the middle trapezius, upper trapezius, lower trapezius and serratus anterior respectively. Hintermeister et al performed an EMG study of the shoulder muscles using elastic band for the resistance during seven exercises. They recommended that shoulder shrug exercises for the upper trapezius muscle, seated

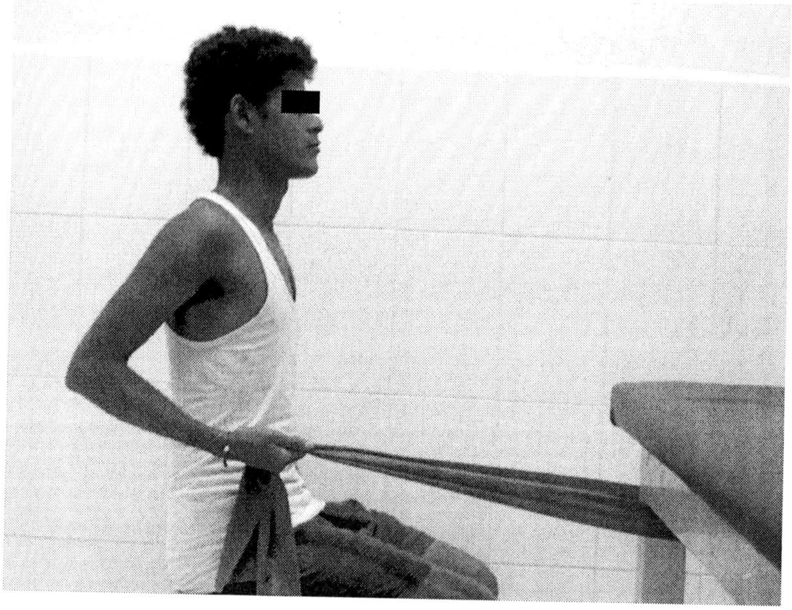

Fig. 3.3: Rowing

rowing exercises for trapezius muscle, forward punch exercise for serratus anterior.

Pushup, dips, flies and bench press are not included in shoulder rehabilitation program as these exercises may increase symptom of shoulder impingement syndrome with AC osteoarthritis.

Researchers have speculated that shorter resting length of pectoralis minor and tightness of posterior capsule are predisposing factors for impingement syndrome. Stretching program may decrease impingement of shoulder. Stretching of anterior and posterior structures of shoulder joint are to be done.

Shoulder rotation by using theraband strengthens external rotators and improves internal rotation range and vice versa (Fig. 3.4).

SURGICAL MANAGEMENT

Acromioplasty

Purpose of the surgery is to decompress the suprahumeral structures.

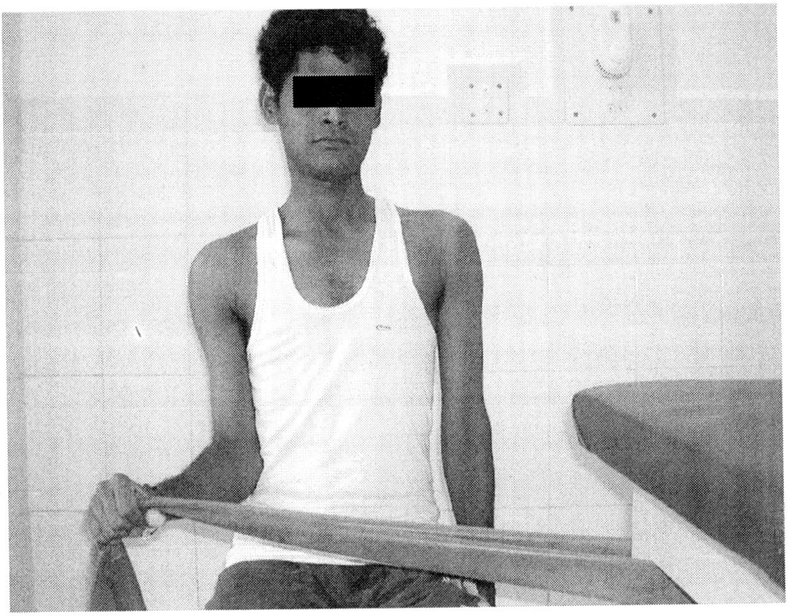

Fig. 3.4: Resisted external rotation and assisted internal rotation using theraband

Indication

Above 30 years when conservative treatment fails.

It can be performed before tendon rupture, where there is excision of anterior 1/3rd of acromion, release of coracoacromial ligament, debridement of thickened degenerated rotator cuff tendon are done.

Distal part of clavicle may be excised in case there is degenerative AC arthritis.

Postoperative physiotherapy

Day 0 → Rest

Day 1 → Relaxed passive flexion and abduction up to 80°.

Before elevation, ensure full external rotation.

After 7-10 days → Elevation through flexion or abduction beyond 80°

Active movement started after 2 weeks, followed by gradual progressive strengthening exercise of rotator cuff to balance deltoid and rotator cuff. The rotator cuffs are already weak and prolonged immobilization may further weaken it.

Open clavicular resection surgical procedure as described by both Gurd and Muford 1941, includes excision of 1–2 cm of distal clavicle and acromion combined. Disadvantage of an open procedure includes the potential injury and resultant weakness in the reattached deltoid and trapezius muscle. The particular complications are much less likely with the arthroscopic technique, as these muscles do not need to be removed and then reattached.

The postoperative complications are inadequate resection, diagnosis errors, joint instability, weakness and miscellaneous factors. Inadequate resection of posterior clavicle allows posterior clavicle to overlap the acromion and is the main cause of residual pain. Joint instability may also be produced if coracoclavicular ligament is released.

Beveling of AC joint is a surgical procedure characterized by excision of protruding osteophytes on under surface of AC joint without resection of distal clavicle. The resection of inferior AC joint's osteophytes results in disruption of inferior AC ligament and capsule, resulting in superior clavicular translation and symptomatic instability.

Supraspinatus Tendon Repair

Anterior acromioplasty and repair of ruptured tendon are done. Transverse repair is preferred over longitudinal as there is more stress in longitudinal.

Transverse incision is given on the skin across the middle of acromion just behind the ACJ. Trapezius and deltoid fibers are splited in the line of their fibers upto the acromion. The acromion is splited with an oscillating saw and retracted to expose the rotator cuff. Identify the ruptured ends of the tendon by internally and externally rotating the shoulder and then end to end anastomosis of tendon is done. Wound is closed layer by layer.

The postoperative resting position is shortened position, i.e. arm rests over an abduction splint or on a pillow for 4–6 weeks as against normal 3 weeks, due to circulatory compromise.

After stitch removal gives passive abduction from abducted resting position in supine lying position for ROM followed by flexion and external rotation. Active ROM started after 6 weeks, to start in gravity eliminated movements followed by antigravity movements. After 8 weeks progressive resisted exercises should be started (Figs 3.5 and 3.6).

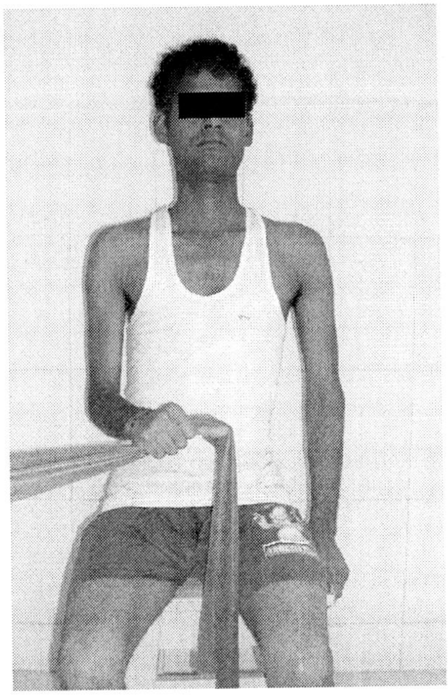

Fig. 3.5: Resisted shoulder internal rotation using theraband to strengthen internal rotators and improve external rotation range

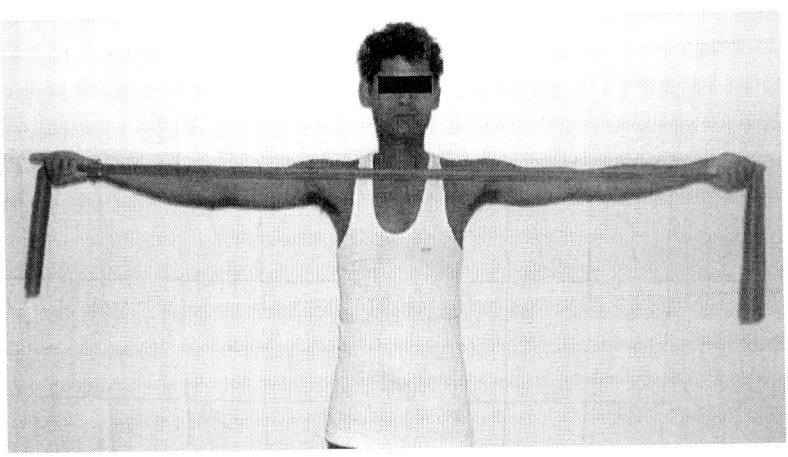

Fig. 3.6: Auto resisted horizontal extension

Adduction below abducted resting position, internal rotation and horizontal adduction shall be avoided for 4-6 week.

Rupture of Biceps Tendon

Degenerative changes occur in various anatomical sites of the shoulder more or less simultaneously as a result of a variety of manual occupations. Comparatively trivial injury may then cause damaged tendons. Degenerative arthritis of ACJ, thickening of coracoacromial ligament impinge the long head of biceps tendon. Associated degenerative changes in the margins of bicipital groove, the tendon undergoes attrition due to longitudinal friction and may rupture spontaneously or from trivial muscle effort.

Rupture of long head of biceps tendon is preceded by chronic shoulder pain and stiffness. At the time of injury there is sharp snap and thereafter pain and sometimes ecchymosis. The ruptured muscle is pulled distally producing typical hollowing in the upper arm and ball-like swelling in the middle arm. There is little loss of power of shoulder flexion, elbow flexion and forearm supination because other muscles can produce near normal power. Since there is no impairment or disability, patient never reports primarily for this problem. It is seen when patient reports with some different problem.

Management

It requires no treatment since it does not give rise to any disability. However, repair may be considered to correct cosmetic disfiguring. The surgical procedure involves either suturing it to bone at the level of the bicipital groove or to the short head of the tendon. In late cases, reassure the patient and no operation is undertaken.

Subacromial Bursitis/Subdeltoid Bursitis

Bursa is a closed cavity present between two structures expected to have friction in between during movement. It is lined by synovium and the synovial fluid keeps the bursal layers moving one over the other eliminating friction.

Subacromial bursitis is not a very common condition of the shoulder joint. It occurs secondary to calcific tendinitis of rotator cuff. Calcific deposit consists of various amorphous calcium salts, primarily calcium apatite in same proportion as in bone. The exact cause is not known, but trauma seems to be one of the precipitating factors. The substance is deposited within the substance of a damaged and relatively avascular supraspinatus tendon. The calcific deposits migrate into the bursa following rupture of degenerated rotator cuff, which forms the floor of the bursa. The onset is always acute, may not present any history of trauma. There is sudden onset of pain within 12–72 hrs. It is always preceded by chronic tendonitis.

Clinical Features

Complaint of intense constant, throbbing type pain.

Patient is worried due to sudden onset of severe pain and holds the hand usually across the chest or by the other hand. There is no arm swing during walking.

Inspection

Swelling present on the lateral aspect of shoulder.

Active Movement

Abduction and elevation is greatly restricted and painful.

Passive Movement

Movements in all directions are restricted in non-capsular pattern with empty end feel. If movements are checked carefully, rotation becomes almost full with the arm by the side. Abduction present up to 60° and flexion up to 90°.

Resisted Isometric Contraction

Patient is hesitant to do the movement. If done carefully, all other movements except abduction are strong and painless.

Palpation

Warm, swelling and tenderness present on the lateral aspect of the shoulder.

Management

Acute Stage

Aim:
- Resolution of acute inflammation
- Prevent further damage

Means:
- Rest to the part by shoulder sling.
- Ice 15- 20 minutes, 5 times/ day.
- To relieve spasm, Inferior Gliding (G1/G2) to head of humerus and/ or Codmann's pendular exercises
  Resolution of acute stage is characterised by absence of rest pain, Abduction ROM improves to 90°

Chronic Stage

Aim:
- Restore mobility
- Prevent recurrence
- Return to activities

Means:
- Thermal dose of US/SWD increases circulation and softens the bursal layers, so applied before mobilization.
- Progressive joint mobilization and muscles strengthening exercises.

OSTEOARTHRITIS OF ACROMIOCLAVICULAR JOINT

Osteoarthritis develops most commonly in absence of known cause of joint degeneration, a condition referred to as primary idiopathic osteoarthritis. It also develops because of injuries, varieties of hereditary inflammatory or developmental, metabolic and neurological disorders, a group of conditions refer to as secondary osteoarthritis. In addition to the disorders responsible for the multiple forms of secondary osteoarthritis, genetic predisposition, obesity, female genders and joint laxity have been identified as risk factors. Risk factors can be classified into two categories. Systemic factors include age, sex, inherited susceptibility osteoarthritis and other factors some of which yet to be identified. Local factors responsible for osteoarthritis are repetitive joint use over decades, joint injury, post-traumatic joint incongruity and instability or malalignment.

The degenerative changes of acromioclavicular joint includes narrowing of the joint space and formation of capsular hypertrophy and inferior osteophyte. It may give rise to impingement syndrome. Capsular pattern of AC joint is restriction at extremes of range of horizontal adduction.

Epidemiology, Prevalence and Incidence

De Palma (1957) dissected 223 sets of acromioclavicular joint from autopsy specimens and found that first regressive changes in acromioclavicular joint in second decade of life. After 50 years, all joints were affected to some degrees. In an analysis of 1000 patients in shoulder pain acromioclavicular abnormalities were found on standard radiograph with prevalency of 12.7%.

Needel, et al examined asymptomatic population by MRI, moderate to severe osteoarthritis of AC joint were found on MRI in 48% of asymptomatic people of age 61 to 88 with incidence doubling after age 80.

In Taft, et al study revealed that 31% of patients who had type III AC joint ligament injury developed osteoarthritis at 10 years follow up. AC joint osteoarthritis may be seen at younger age in sports like tennis, swimming and pitching.

Clinical Features

Pain

Night pain is typical, and day time pain is related to overhead activity. The presenting complaint of pain is not usually localized to AC joint, but patient commonly presents with a dull ache involving the deltoid area. AC osteoarthritis has a painful arc between 120° to 180° whereas rotator cuff impingement has pain at range of 60° to 120°. Local tenderness present.

Provocative Tests

Several tests like local tenderness at joint, the active compression test (O'Brien sign), cross-arm adduction and Paxino's sign have been developed for physical examination of acromial clavicular joint and also 2% lidocaine injection test used for isolation of AC joint osteoarthritis.

Injection Test

0.5 ml omnipaque 240 lohexol, 240 mg/ml is injected into AC joint by a 25-gauge, 1.5 inch needle. Then 1 ml of 2% lidocaine is injected. This causes relief of pain when impingement sign is repeated.

Diagnostic Imaging

Radiograph

Plain radiographs were evaluated for any abnormalities of AC joint, including joint space narrowing, marginal osteophytes or subchondral cysts. Zenca view is particularly helpful for evaluating AC joint pathology. This view allows an unobstructed view of the joint and inferior osteophytes. Axial view is recommended for os acromiale.

Magnetic Resonance Imaging

It can detect capsular hypertrophy, effusions, subchondral edema and an os acromiale.

Bone scans: Bone scanning is the best imaging modality for the diagnosis of AC joint pain. When Paxino's sign and bone scanning are both positive, the diagnosis of AC joint pain is virtually certain.

Management

Non-steroidal anti-inflammatory drugs (NSAIDS) are frequently prescribed, but they have significant side effects. Cyclooxygenase 2 - selective inhibitors (Coxibs) were initially thought to be safer alternative to NSAIDS, but recent concerns have included gastrointestinal, cardiovascular, renal, and hepatic side effects.

Hot-pack and ultrasound have little therapeutic value. Benefits have been reported with manual therapy technique used in combined joint mobility, stretching exercises and strengthening exercise. Manipulation therapy treatments like Maitland, Mulligan and Kaltenborn have been advocated for AC joint. Maitland and Kaltenborn recommended PA and caudal glide of lateral end of clavicle for AC joint mobilization, whereas Mulligan suggests that the sustained inferior glide of lateral end of clavicle with active abduction-elevation movement relieves pain at the AC joint and PA glide with horizontal flexion extension is also helpful.

The mechanism by which manual therapy exerts its ameliorative effects in clinical practices remains to be fully elucidated. A number of studies have shown that spinal manipulative therapy evokes a specific hypoalgesic effect. Manipulation induced hypoalgesia appears to be non-opioid in nature, that is it is not reversed by naloxene and does not develop tolerance to repeated stimulations. Manual therapy produces mechanical hypoalgesia rather than thermal hypoalgesia in both symptomatic and asymptomatic study population. Mobilization stimulates articular mechanoreceptors exerting a reciprocally coordinated reflexogenic influence on the muscle tone and excitability of stretch reflex in all striated muscle. It also produces pre-synaptic inhibition of nociceptive afferent transmission through synapses in basal spinal nucleus of spinal cord and activating descending pathway from dorsal periaqueductal gray or d PAG, thereby reducing pain. It has also been hypothesized that the manual therapy mechanically stretches shortened collaginous tissue and improves interstitial fluid control. It causes a physiological loading and unloading of joint cartilage, which facilitates the flow of synovial fluid within in the joint, ensuring adequate nutrition for the articular cartilage.

BIBLIOGRAPHY

1. Abbot JH. Mobilization with movement applied to the elbow affects shoulder range of movement in subjects with lateral epicondylgia. Manual therapy 2001;6(3):170-7.
2. Altman RD. Osteoarthritis. Aggravating factors and therapeutic measures. Postgraduate Medicine 1986;80:150-63.
3. Anderson L, Rush R, et al. The effects of a thera-band exercise programme on shoulder internal rotation strength. Phy Ther 1992; 72:S40 (suppl).
4. Antonaci F, Sand T, et al. Pressure algometry in healthy subjects: Inter-examiner variability. Scand J Rehab 1998;30:3-8.
5. Atkins CJ, Ziellinski A. An electronic method for measuring joint tender in rheumatoid arthritis. Arthritis and rheumatism 1992;4: 407-10.
6. Bang MD, Deyel GD. Comparison of supervised exercise with and without manual therapy for patient with shoulder impingement syndrome. J OrthoP Sports Phys Ther 2000;30:126-32.
7. Bannister GC, Wallace WA, Stableforth PG, et al. The management of acute acromioclavicular dislocation. J Bone Joint Surg 1989; 71B(5):848-50.
8. Beeton KS. Manual therapy master class: The peripheral joints. Churchill Livingstone. Peripheral mobilization with movement: 129-44.
9. Bengtsson M, Lunsjo K, Hamadsson Y, et al. High patient satisfaction after arthroscopic subacromial decompression for shoulder impingement. Acta Orthopaedica 2006;71(1):138-42.
10. Bigliani Lu and Levine WN. Subacromial impingement syndrome. J Bone Joint Surg Am 1997;79:1854-68.
11. Bohannon RW, Lusardi MM. Modified sphygmomanometer versus strain gauge hand-held dynamometer. Arch Phys Med Rehabil 1991;72:911-4.
12. Bonsell S, Pearsall AW, Heitman RJ, et al. The relationship of age, gender, and degenerative changes observed on radiographs of the shoulder in asymptomatic individuals. J Bone Joint Surg 2000; 82B:1135-9.
13. Borstad Jd, Ludeing MP. The effect of long versus short pectoris minor resting length on shoulder kinematics in healthy individuals. J Orthop Sports Phys Ther 2005;35:227-38.

14. Brox JI, Staff PH, Ljuggren AE, Brevik JI, Arthroscopy surgery compared with supervised exercises in patients with rotator cuff disease (Stage-II impingement syndrome). Br Med J. 1993;307: 899-903.
15. Bucherger DJ. Introduction of a new physical examination procedure for the differentiation of AC joint lesions and sub-acronomial impingement. J Manipulative Physiol Ther 1999;22: 316-21.
16. Bulgen Dy, Binder A, Hazelman BL. Immunological studies in frozen shoulder. J. Rheumatol 1982;9:893-8.
17. Buttaci C, Stitik TP, Yonclass PP, Foye PM. Osteoarthritis of acromioclavicular joint. A review of anatomy, biomechanics, diagnosis and treatment. AM J Phys Med Rehabil 2004;83:791-7.
18. Byl NN, Melnick M. The neural consequences of repetition: Clinical implication of a learning hypothesis. J Hand Ther 1997;10:160-74.
19. Calvart PT. Clinical examination of the shoulder. Incopelands, (Ed) Shoulder surgery. 1st Edn WB Saunders Company Ltd, London, P 1-14.
20. Chaitow L. Muscle energy techniques, 2nd edn. Churchill Livingstone Edinburgh: 2001.
21. Chard MD, Hazleman BL, King RH, Reiss BB. Shoulder disorders in the elderly: a community survey. Arthritis Rheum 1991;34:766-9.
22. Chen AL, Rokito AS, Zuckerman JD. The role of the acromioclavicular joint in impingement syndrome. Clin in Sports Med 2003;22:343-57.
23. Christopher SO. How manipulation works. The Journal of the Hong Kong Physiotherapy Association 1986;8:30-4.
24. Chronopoulus E, Kim TK, Park HD, et al. Diagnostic value of physical tests for isolated chronic acromioclavicular lesions. Am J Sports Med. 2004;32:655-61.
25. Coroy and Hayes KU.The effect of joint mobilization as a component of comprehensive treatment for primary shoulder impingement syndrome. J Orthop Sports Phy Ther 1998;28:3-14.
26. Cuomo F, Kummer FJ, Zuckerman JD, et al. The influence of acromioclavicular joint morphologic on rotator cuff tear. J Shoulder Elbow Surg 1998;7:555-9.
27. Dalu J, Oboziv. The influence of distal clavicular resection and rotator cuff repair on the effectiveness of anterior acromioplasty. Clin Orthop. 1989;247:117-23.
28. David TF. Risk factors of osteoarthritis. J Orthop Res 2004;427:S 16-S21 (supplement).
29. Debaski RE, Parsons IM, woo SL-Y, et al. Effect of capsular injury on acromioclavicular joint mechanics. Bone Joint Surg 2001;83A: 1344-51.

30. Deyle GD, et al. Physical therapy treatment effectiveness for osteoarthritis of knee: A randomized comparison of supervised clinical exercise and manual therapy procedures versus a home exercise programme. Phys Ther 2005;85:1301-17.
31. Dodd KJ. Strength training for older people in; Morrish schoo A: optimizing exercise and physical activity in older people. Butterworth, 125-52.
32. Donatelli RA. Impingement syndrome and impingement related instability. Physical therapy of the shoulder. Churchill Livingston 1997;229-56.
33. Edelson JG, Zuckerman J, Hershkovitz I. Os acromiale: anatomy and surgical implications. J Bone Joint Surg 1992;74B:589-94.
34. Ekstrom RA, Donatelli RA, et al. Surface electromyographic analysis of exercises for the trapezius and serratus anterior muscles. J Orthop Sports Phys Ther 2003;33:247-58.
35. Ernberg LA, Potter HG. Radiographic evaluation of the acromioclavicular and sternoclavicular joint. Clin Sport Med 2003;22:255-75.
36. Frost P and Anderson JH. Shoulder impingement syndrome in relation to shoulder intensive work. Occup Environ Med 1999; 56:494-8.
37. Frost P, Anderson JH. Shoulder impingement syndrome in relation to shoulder intensive work. Occu P Environ Med 1999;56:494-8.
38. Fu FH, Hanner CD, Klein AH. Shoulder impingement syndrome - A critical review. Clin Ortho P 1991;269:162-73.
39. G Leviseth, et al. Changes in muscles fiber cross sectional area and concentrations of Na, K- ATPase in deltoid muscle in patients with impingement syndrome. J Orthop Sports Phys Ther, 1994; 19:146-56.
40. Gartsman GM. Acromioclavicular joint resection. Am J Sports Med 1991;19:2-5.
41. Gillars, et al. Neurologic basis of manual medicine. Physical medicine and rehabilitation clinic of North America 1996;4:693-713.
42. Glousman RE, Jobe F, Tibove J, Moynes D, Antonelli D, Perrys J. Dynamic electromyography analysis of the throwing shoulder with glenohumeral instability. J Bone Joint Surg. 1988;70-A:220-6.
43. Glousman RE. Instability versus impingement syndrome in throwing athlete. Ortho P Clin North Am 1993;24:89-99.
44. Green-field B, Catlin PA, Coats PW, Green E, Mc Donald JJ, North C. Posture in-patient with shoulder over use injuries and healthy individuals. J Ortho P Sports Phys Ther 1995;21:287-95.
45. Gurbuz H, Unalan H, Saltik HS, et al. The role of acromioclavicular arthritis in impingement syndromes. Yonsei Medical Journal1998; 39:97-102.

46. Haarhr JP, Osteogard S, et al. Arthroscopic decompression and physiotherapy have similar effectiveness for subacromial impingement. J Bone Joint Surg 2005;87:2595.
47. Helwa A, Goldsmith CH, Smythe HA. Modified sphygmomanometer - Instrument to measure muscle strength. Validation study. J Chronic Dis. 1981;34:353-61.
48. Helwa A, Goldsmith CH, Symthe HA. Patient observer and instrument variation in the measurement of strength of shoulder abductors muscles in patients with rheumatoid arthritis using a modified sphygmomanometer. J Rheumatol 1986;13(6):1044-9.
49. Hertel R, Windisch W, Schuster A, Balmar FT. Transacromial approach to obtain fusion of unstable os acromial. J Shoulder Elbow Surg 1998;7:606-9.
50. Hintermeister RA, Lange GW, Schultheis JM, Bey MS, Hawkin RS. Electromyographic activity and applied load during shoulder rehabilitation exercises using elastic resistance. Am J Sports Med 1998;26(2):210-20.
51. Hisch C-Y, Vicenzino B, et al. Mulligan's mobilization with movement for the thumb: a single case report using magnetic resonance imaging to evaluate the positional fault hypothesis. Manual therapy 2002;7(1):44-9.
52. Hogewag JA, Lingerie MJ, et al. Algometry: Measuring pain threshold: Method and characteristics in healthy subjects. Scand J Rehabi 1992;24:99-103.
53. Holloway GB, Schenk T, William GR, Ramsev ML, Lannotti JP. Arthroscopy capsular release for the treatment of refractory post-operative or postfracture shoulder stiffness. J Bone Joint Surg. Am 2001, 83.1682-7.
54. Hughes CJ, Hurd K, et al. Resistance properties of thera-band tubing during shoulder abduction exercise. J Orthop Sports PhysTher 1999;29:413-20.
55. Huskissn EC, Hart FD. Pain threshold and arthritis. British Medical Journal 1972;4:193-5.
56. Jacobsson L, Lindgarde F, Mantherpe R. The common Rheumatic complaint over a six-week duration in a twelve months period in defined Swedish population: Prevalence and relationships. Scand J Rheumatol 1989;18:353-60.
57. Jensen K, Anderson HO, et al. Pressure-pain threshold in human temporal region: Evaluation of a new pressure algometer. Pain 1986;25:313-23.
58. John CL, Russell F, Warren, Margaret GE. A self-administered questionnaire for assessment of symptoms and function of the shoulder. J Bone Joint Surg. 1997;79-A:738-48.

59. Kaegi C, Thibault MC, et al. The interrater reliability of force measurement using modified sphygmomanometer in elderly subjects. Phys Ther 1998;1095-103.
60. Kamkar R, Irrgang JJ, Whiteney SL. Non-operative management of secondary shoulder impingement syndrome. J Orthop Sport Phy Ther 1993;17:212-4.
61. Kapanji IA. The physiology of the joint. 5th Edn. Churchil Livingstone. Volume 1, 1-70.
62. Kessel L, Watson M. The painful arc syndrome. J Bone Joint Surg 1977;59B:166-71.
63. Kosek E, Ekholm J, et al. A comparison of pressure pain threshold in different tissues and body regions: Long-term reliability of pressure algometer in healthy volunteers. Scand J Rehab med 1993;25:117-24.
64. Langley GB, et al. A simple pressure dolorimeter for the quantification of joint tenderness in inflammatory arthritis. Rheumatol lnt 1993;3:109-12.
65. Lee KW, Dabaski RE, Chen CH, et al. Functional evaluation of the ligament at acromioclavicular joint during antero-posterior and superoinferior translation. Am J Sports Med 1997;25:858-62.
66. Leroux JL, codine P, Thomas E, Pcholle M, Maithe D, Blotman F. Isokinetic evaluation of rotational strength in normal shoulders and shoulders with impingement syndrome. Clin Ortho P 1994; 304:108-15. (Abstract).
67. Lori A, Michener, Mathew K, Walsworth Evie N, Burnet. Effectiveness of rehabilitation for patient with subacromial impingement syndrome. J Hand Ther 2004;17:152-64.
68. Loudon J, Bell S, and Johnston J. The clinical orthopedic assessment guide of human kinetics; 1998:69-91.
69. Ludewig MP and Borstad JD. Effects of a home exercise programme on the shoulder pain and functional status in construction workers. Occu Environ Med 2003;60:841-9.
70. Ludiwig PM, Cook TM. Nawoczinski DA. Three dimensional scapular orientation and muscle activity at selected positions of humeral elevation. J Orthop Sports Phys Ther 1996;24:57-65.
71. Ludiwing PM, Cook TM. Alterations in shoulder kinematics and associated muscle activity in people with symptoms of shoulder impingement. Phy Ther 2000;80:276-91.
72. Mahakkunu KP, Surin P. Prevalence of osteophytes associated with the acromion and acromioclavicular joint. Clin Anat 2003;16: 506-10.
73. Maitland GD. Peripheral manipulation; 3rd Boston, mass; Butter worth- Heineman 1991;157-9.

74. Mcclure, et al. Shoulder function and 3-dimensional kinematics in people with shoulder impingement syndrome before and after 6-week programme. Phys Ther 2004;84:834-48.
75. Merskey H and Spear FG. The reliability of the pressure algometer. British J Soc Clin Psychol. 1964;3:130-6.
76. Mikesky AE, Topp R, Wiglesworth JK, et al. Efficacy of a home-based training programme for older adult using elastic tubing. Eur J Apply Physiol. 1994;69:316-20.
77. Montellese P, Dancy T. The acromioclavicular joint. Prim Care Clin Office Pract 2004;31:857-66.
78. Morrison DS, Grenbaum BS, Einhorn A. Shoulder impingement. Ortho Clin North Am 2000;31:285-93.
79. Morrisson DS, Frogameni AD and Woodworth P. Non-operative treatment of subacromial impingement syndrome. J Bone Joint 1997;79A:732-7.
80. Moskowitz RW, et al. Osteoarthritis; 3rd edn. WB Saunders Company: Upper extremity consideration. Shoulder; 469-77.
81. Mosley JB, Jobe FW, Pink M, Perry J, Tibore J. EMG analysis of scapular muscles during a shoulder rehabilitation programme. Am J Sports Med. 1992;20:128-34.
82. Mulligan BR. Manual therapy. 3rd edition 1995;124.
83. Needell SD, Zlatkin MB, Sher JS, et al. MRI imaging of the rotator cuff: Peritendinous and bone abnormalities in an asymptomatic population. AJR 1996;166:863-7.
84. Neer CS. Anterior acromioplasty for the chronic impingement syndrome in the shoulder. J Bone Joint Surg 1972;54A:41-50.
85. Neuman DA. Kinesiology of the musculoskeletal system. 1st edn Mosby 2002.
86. Ogata S and Uhthoff HK. Acromial enthesopathy and rotator cuff tear. A radiologic and histologic postmortem investigation of the coracoacromial arch. Clin Orthop 1990;2:39-48.
87. Oppenheimer A. Arthritis of the acromioclavicular joint. J Bone Joint Surg 1943;4:867-70.
88. Park HB, Yokoth A, Gill HS, et al. Diagnostic accuracy of clinical tests for the different degrees of subacromial impingement syndrome. J Bone Joint Surg 2005;87A:1446-54.
89. Patterson RM, Stegink Jansen CW, et al. Material properties of thera-band tubing. Phys Ther 2001;82:1437-45.
90. Peterson CJ. Degeneration of the acromioclavicular joint. Acta OrthoP Scand 1983;54:434-8.
91. Petersson CJ, Redlund-Johnell I. Radiographic joint space in normal acromioclavicular joints. Acta Orthop Scand 1983;54:431-3.
92. Phil page. Thera-band tubing. Phys Ther 2002;82:191-2.

93. Philadelphia panel evidence-based clinical practice guidelines on selected rehabilitation interventions for shoulder pain. Phys Ther 2001;81:1719-30.
94. Picavet HS, Schouten JS. Musculoskeletal pain in the Netherlands: Prevalence, consequences and risk groups, the DMC (3) - Study: Pain 2003;102:167-78.
95. Pink MM, Tibone JE. The painful shoulder in the swimming athletes. Ortho Clin North Am 2000;30:247-61.
96. Price D, MC Grath, et al. The validation of visual analogue scale as ratio scale measures for chronic and experimental pain. 1983;17:45-56.
97. Proicevic et al. Rotator cuff impingement. J Manipulative Physiol Ther 2005;580-90.
98. Ranfree KJ, Wright TW. Anatomy and biomechanics of acromioclavicular and sternoclavicular joint. Clin Sports Med 2003; 22:219-37.
99. Razmjou H, Holtby R, Myhr T. Pain provocative shoulder tests. Reliability and validity of the impingement tests. Physiotherapy Can 2004;56:229-36.
100. Reinold MM, et al. Electromyographic analysis of rotator cuff and deltoid musculature during common shoulder external rotation exercises. J Orthop Sports Phys Ther 2004;34:385-94.
101. Renfree KJ, Wright TW. Anatomy and biomechanics of the acromioclavicular joint and sternoclavicular joint. Clin Sports Med 2003;22:219-37.
102. Revill S, Robinson J, et al. The reliability of a linear analogue for evaluating pain. Anesthesia. 1976;31:1191-8.
103. Rice CL, Cunningham DA, et al. Strength in an elderly population. Arch Phys Med Rehabil 1989;70:391-7.
104. Robert S, Gailey JR and Michele AR. Manual Modalities: Physiological basis of rehabilitation medicine, 3rd edn-2001;761-73.
105. Rockwood CA, Witham GR, Young DC. Disorder of the acromioclavicular joint. In: Rockwood Jr CA, Mattason FA (Editors). The shoulder, 2nd edition, Philadelphia: WB Saunders; 1988;483-553.
106. Rudzki JR, Matava MJ, Paletta GA. Complications of treatment of acromioclavicular and sternoclavicular joint injuries. Clin Sports Med 2003;22:387-405.
107. Schmitt L, Synder - Mackler L. Role of scapular stabilizer in etiology and treatment of impingement syndrome. J Orthop sports Phy ther 1999;29:31-8.
108. Scovazzo ML, Browne A, Pink, et al. The painful shoulder during freestyle swimming: An electromyographic cinematographic analysis of twelve muscles. Am J Sports Med. 1991;19:577-82.

109. Soslowsky LJ, Thmopoulus S, Tun S, et al. Overuse activity injuries of the supraspinatus tendon in an anatomical model. A histological and biomechanical study. J Shoulder Elbow Surg 2000;9:78-84 (abstract).
110. Steinfield R, Stuart M. A common sense approach to shoulder problems; Mayo Clinic Prac 1999;74:785-94.
111. Stenlund B, Goldie I, Hagberg M, et al. Radiographic osteoarthrosis in the acromioclavicular joint resulting from manual work or exposure to vibration. Br Ind Med 1992;49:588-93.
112. Stenlund B. Shoulder tendonitis and osteoarthritis of the acromioclavicular joint in relation to sports. Br J Sport Med 1993; 27:125-30.
113. Strobel, et al. MRI feature of the acromioclavicular joint that predicts pain relief from intra-articular injection. AJR; 180:755-60.
114. Struhls. Anterior internal impingement: an arthroscopic observation. Arthroscopy 2002;18:2-7.
115. Taft TN, Wilson FC, Oglesby JW. Dislocation of the acromioclavicular joint. J Bone Joint Surg Am 1987;69:1045-51.
116. Takeda Y, Kashiwanguchis, Endo K, Matsura T, Sesa T. The most effective exercise for strengthening the supraspinatus muscle.: evaluation by magnetic resonance imaging. Am J Sports Med 2002;30:374-81.
117. Therel Keld AJ. The effect of manual therapy on connective tissue. Phy Ther 1992;72:893-902.
118. Tim Lu, et al. Motion analysis: Shoulder mechanics mobilize joint movement. Biomechanics 2000 Nov. (Rehab supplement).
119. Townsend H, Jobe FW, Pink M, Perry J. Electromyographic analysis of the glenohumeral muscles during a baseball rehabilitation programme. Am J sports Med. 1999;19:264-71.
120. Tyler TF, Nahow RC, Nicholas SJ, et al. Quantifying shoulder rotation weakness in patients with shoulder impingement. J Shoulder Elbow Surg 2005;14:570-4.
121. Tyuina TV. Age-related characteristics of the human acromioclavicular joint. Arkh Anat Gistol Embriol 1985;89:75-81.
122. Urwin M, Symmons D, and Allison T, et al. Estimating the burden of musculoskeletal disorders in the community the comparative prevalence of symptoms at different anatomical sites, and the relation to social deprivation. Ann Rheum Dis. 1998;57:649-55.
123. Uzaki J, Fujimoto, Nagawa Y, Masuhara K, and Tamai S. Tear of the rotator cuff of the shoulder associated with pathological changes in the acromion. A study in cadaver. J Bone Joint Surg 1988;70:1224-34.

124. Vander Windt DA, Koes BW, de Jong BA, Bouter IM. Shoulder disorders in general practices. Incidence, patient characteristics, and management. Ann Rheum Dis 1995;54:959-64.
125. Vatainen U, Pirinen A, Makela A. Radiological evaluation of the acromioclavicular joint. Skeletal Radiolog1991;20:115-6.
126. Vechio P. Kavangagh R, Hazleman BL, King RH. Shoulder pain in a community - based rheumatology clinic. Br J Rheumatol. 1995; 34:440-2.
127. Vicenzino B, Paugmali A, Baratoski S and Wright A. Specific manipulative therapy treatment for chronic lateral epicondylagia produces uniquely characteristic hypoalgesia. Manual therapy 2001;6(4):205-12.
128. Vicenzino B. Lateral epicondylalgia: A musculoskeletal physiotherapy perspective. Manual therapy 2003;8(2):66-79.
129. Walton J, Mahajan S, Paxinos A, Marshal J, Murrell GA. Diagnostic value of tests for AC joint Pain. J Bone Joint Surg Am 2004;86:807-12.
130. Warrer JP, Micheli, Arslanian L, Kenedy J, Kennedy R. Patterns of flexibility, laxicity and strength in normal shoulders with instability and impingement. Am J Sports Med. 1990;18:366-74.
131. Wing KC. Shoulder impingement syndrome. Phys Med Rehabil Clin N Am 2004;15:493-510.
132. Worecester JN, Green DP. Osteoarthritis of the acromioclavicular joint. Clin OrthoP 1968;69:69-73.
133. Wucker N, Plitz W, Roetman B. Biomechanical data concerning the shoulder impingement syndrome. Clin Orthop Rel Res 1994;5: 242-9.
134. Wyke BD, Polacek P. Articular neurology. The present proposition. J Bone Joint Surg 1975;57-B.401.

Chapter 4

Adhesive Capsulitis

Adhesive capsulitis was first described in 1872 by Duplay and named frozen shoulder by Codman in 1934. The term "frozen shoulder" is defined as a clinical condition with restricted active and passive range of motion (ROM) in all directions, including flexion, abduction, and rotation.

Adhesive capsulitis is a condition of glenohumeral joint, in which there is restriction of active and passive ROM in capsular pattern, i.e. external rotation and abduction are mostly restricted followed by internal rotation and flexion whereas extension is relatively free.

Naviaser (1945) dissected 63 shoulders postmortem with limited movement on clinical examination and found that the capsule of the shoulder joint was tight, closely applied to the head of humerus and gaped widely when incised anteriorly. Limitation of abduction was due to adhesion between two capsular surfaces inferiorly. He suggested adhesive capsulitis, characterized by thickening and contracture of capsule which microscopically showed to be the site of reparative inflammatory change.

Viessel (1949) carried out arthrography and found obliteration of inferior redundant capsular fold of glenohumeral joint due to adhesion, anterior joint capsule along with subscapular bursa, were obliterated more than posterior joint capsule. Obliteration of biceps sheath space seen.

Reeves (1966) found a marked reduction of the volume of the fluid that was injectable at constant pressure in arthritic shoulder, less so when the lesion follows trauma.

Reduction of anterior joint capsule space indicates tightness of anterior capsule limiting shoulder external rotation most. Reduction of inferior redundant joint capsular fold limits shoulder abduction. Relatively less reduction of posterior joint capsule space indicates tightness of posterior capsule limiting shoulder internal rotation to lesser extent.

Cyriax's selective tissue tension test reveals negative response to resisted isometric contraction indicating no contractile tissue (muscle) involvement. Limitation of shoulder movements in capsular pattern, i.e. ER would be more limited than abduction, which would be more limited than IR is suggestive of tightness of joint capsule.

X-ray shows no bony abnormally except disuse osteoporosis.

In 1969, Lundberg categorized the frozen shoulder into idiopathic or primary adhesive capsulitis and secondary adhesive capsulitis. The pathogenesis of the idiopathic form remains unclear, although there are many proposed mechanisms.

A definition of frozen shoulder was presented by **Reeves in 1975**, who has called it "an idiopathic condition of the shoulder characterized by the spontaneous onset of pain in the shoulder with restriction of movement in every direction".

In 1994, Zuckerman proposed a classification schema where primary frozen shoulder and idiopathic adhesive capsulitis are considered identical and not associated with a systemic condition or history of injury. **Harryman and Neviaser** suggested endocrine, immunologic, inflammatory, and biochemical changes as possible causes. **Janda** described how there is an increased incidence in patients with diabetes. Secondary adhesive capsulitis develops when there is a known intrinsic, extrinsic, or systemic cause.

In 2002, Cleland and Durall described **Adhesive capsulitis**—a disorder of the glenohumeral joint of unknown etiology which is characterized by painful and gradually progressive restriction of active and passive glenohumeral joint motion. Such disorders tend to run a long and protracted course and eventually become self-limiting.

According to **Nakagawa OY, Kurai** Pathoanatomy shows decreased volume of the glenohumeral joint with restricted ROM. The arthroscopic examination shows a reduced volume with a tight capsule, synovial hypertrophy, and neovascular proliferation. In the **first stage or freezing stage**, the early inflammatory stage, hypervascular synovitis is seen. In the **second stage or frozen stage**, there is a decrease in hypervascularity and synovitis; however, capsular contraction and thickening is noted on arthroscopic evaluation.

In the **third stage or thawing phase**, no synovitis is seen, and there is a decrease in the thickness of the capsule. Arthroscopy is rarely indicated in the first or third stage of adhesive capsulitis. Although the glenohumeral joint synovial capsule is involved, much of the disease process involves structures outside the shoulder joint, including the coracohumeral ligament, rotator interval, **subscapularis musculotendinous unit**, and the subacromial bursae.

EPIDEMIOLOGY

According to the American Academy of Orthopedic Surgeons, it ranks as the third most common musculoskeletal complaint behind knee and spinal disorders (**James Camarinos 2009**). Frozen shoulder is felt to have a prevalence rate of 2% in the general population; however, an 11% prevalence rate is reported in diabetics. Patients with type I diabetes have a 40% chance of developing a frozen shoulder in their lifetimes. Frozen shoulder might affect both shoulders in up to 16% of patients; however, a relapse is uncommon. Adhesive capsulitis is more common in the fifth and sixth decades of life, and other medical problems should be investigated in patients below 40 years of age. Women are affected more than men with a ratio of 58:42. **(Thierry D 2005).**

ETIOLOGY

- Exact cause not known
- Females are more affected than male with 2:1 ratio, and elderly above 40 years of age are more affected than young, except diabetic patients. More commonly, it involves nondominant shoulder and in about 12% cases it is bilateral. The followings are probable hypothesis:

Pain and Immobilization

Patient does not or cannot move the part due to pain. The proliferated collagen fibers develop into thick and short scar tissue interfering with movements.

Posture

Head forward posture, increased thoracic kyphosis and rounded shoulder disturb normal upward orientation of glenoid fossa of scapula, which leads to loss of tension of superior joint capsule and coracohumeral ligament. Overactivity of rotator cuff increases tensile stress over the capsular ligament to which the rotator cuff tendons blend. The chronic inflammation thickens and fibroses the capsule over time.

Periarthritic Personality (Anxious Person)

Anxiety changes the posture to kyphotic and reduces the pain threshold, so in some minor problems they voluntarily restrict the movements.

Degenerative

As it occurs more in elderly persons, it is thought to be degenerative. As it occurs more in female and particularly postmenopausal women, so some postmenopausal factors may be responsible.

Incidence of Periarthritis is more in Diabetics

Secondary frozen shoulder develops due to pain or immobilization following trauma or surgery. In the absence of any known factor the condition is classified as primary idiopathic frozen shoulder. Primary frozen shoulder is the most common form and thought to be autoimmune disorder.

REEV CLASSIFICATION (3 STAGES)

Stage I lasts from 3 months to 9 months. Characterized by pains.

Gradual reduction of joint volume with obliteration of subscapular bursa space, sometimes bicipital sheath space develops.

At end of stage I, there is reduction in intensity of pain and stiffness develops.

Stage-II lasts from 4–12 months. Characterized by stiffness. Patient complaints of pain during activities due to stiffness.

Stage-III lasts from 5 months to 2 years. It is the stage of spontaneous recovery. According to REEV, it is a self-limiting condition. The movement which is restricted first recovers first, i.e. there is gradual return of external rotation with reappearance of subscapularis bursa. Next abduction followed by internal rotation recovers.

Duration of painful period is directly proportional to duration of recovery. If painful period is shorter, fast recovery occurs whereas when painful period is longer, recovery becomes late.

CYRIAX CLASSIFICATION (3 STAGES)

Stage-I: Patient complaints of pain on the lateral brachial region, not extending below the elbow. Patient can lie on the affected side shoulder.

Movements are restricted in capsular pattern with elastic end-feel because of muscle spasm. Pain is experienced at the end range of movements and activities.

Stage-II: Patient complains of pain on the lateral brachial region and unable to lie on the affected side shoulder.
Some criteria of stage I could be present.

Stage-III: Severe pain extending below the elbow. Pain at rest, becomes more in the night. Patient cannot lie on the affected side shoulder, lying on the affected shoulder becomes painful due to stretching/compression of involved structures. Movements restricted in capsular pattern with leathery end feel because of the tension of tight capsule.

CONVENTIONAL CLASSIFICATION

Acute stage is characterized by pain on lateral brachial region, more in the night. Restriction of ROM due to pain and spasm.

Chronic stage is characterized by absence of rest pain and night pain. Pain becomes localized only in lateral brachial region. Pain experienced during activities due to stretching of tight joint capsule. Movements restricted in capsular pattern with leathery end feel.

CLINICAL FEATURES

History

Mode of Onset: Gradual onset of pain and restriction of movements.

Patient may present the history of trauma/immobilization or painful shoulder condition. Diabetes may be present.

Pain: Patient complains of vague dull aching pain over lateral brachial region (C5, C6).

Finds inability/difficulty to do overhead activities like combing, dressing and undressing, etc., due to limitation of external rotation abduction. Reaching the back pocket or tying the dhoti or saree, fastening bra, etc. become difficult due to limitation of internal rotation.

Observation

Posture: Increased thoracic/cervico-thoracic kyphosis, head forward and rounded shoulder (protracted and depressed).

Facial Appearance: Anxious

Attitude of the upper extremity: Arm by the side or across the chest, inadequate arm swing during walking.

Inspection

Skin: Not contributory.

Soft tissue: Disuse atrophy of both periscapular and shoulder girdle muscles present.

Bony: Head forward, increased thoracic/cervicothoracic kyphosis, rounded shoulders with protraction and depression of scapulae.

Movements

Active Movements

Willingness of the patient to move: in acute painful condition one finds difficult to move the arm.

Pain: Acute condition, pain and spasm restrict the movement. Pain experienced throughout the abduction elevation movements.
Chronic condition, pain experienced at the end range of existing limited abduction elevation movement due to stretching of tight capsule.

ROM: Restricted in capsular pattern, i.e. external rotation and abduction restricted more, and internal rotation and flexion restricted to lesser extent.

Painful arc: Pain may be present during mid-range of abduction-elevation.

Passive Movements

ROM: Restricted in capsular pattern with muscle spasm end feels at acute stage and leathery end feels at chronic stage.

Pain: Acute condition, pain experienced throughout the abduction elevation movements.

Chronic condition, pain experienced at the end range of existing limited abduction elevation movement due to stretching of tight capsule.

Painful arc may be present at the midrange of abduction-elevation.

End feel: Acute stage, muscle spasm end feel with pain encountered before the motion barrier. Chronic stage, leathery end feel with pain encountered after the motion barrier.

Joint play: Amplitude of joint play restricted in the following order with pain:

- Posterior to anterior gliding of head of humerus is restricted more limiting the external rotation most
- Inferior gliding restricted limiting abduction
- Posterior gliding restricted limiting internal rotation.

Resisted Isometric Contraction

Muscle strength could be reduced because of disuse atrophy due to pain and stiffness, but no pain experienced during resisted isometric contraction against maximum resistance.

Neuromuscular examination:

Some weakness may be present due to disuse atrophy. No other neurological impairment present.

Palpation

- *Skin:* Nothing contributory
- *Soft tissue:* Tenderness may be present over insertion of rotator cuff at greater tuberosity, long head of biceps at bicipital groove
- *Bony:* Greater tuberosity, acromion, AC joint, SC joint.

MANAGEMENT

Acute Stage

Acute stage is characterized by pain at rest and restriction of motion with muscle spasm end feel.

Aim

- To relieve pain and spasm
- Prevent and correct stiffness

- Prevent disuse atrophy
- Correct posture

Means

a. Apply ice for 15–20 minutes, 5 times per day
b. Following ice therapy, apply Grade I or II inferior gliding of head of humerus. Oscillatory, rhythmic Grade I/II mobilization reduces spasm and relieves the pain.

   Muscle spasm pulls the head of humerus upward, which gets impinged against coracoacromial arch giving rise to pain and spasm. Inferior gliding relieves pain by correcting impingement and thereby reduces the spasm.
c. Pendular shoulder movements (Codman's exercise):
   Stand leaning against a table by the sound hand, swing the affected arm forward-backward for flexion-extension, sideway for abduction-adduction and clockwise- anticlockwise for rotation and circumduction. One can hold a dumb-bell, which will apply inferior gliding, while doing the exercise.
d. Postural correction:
   - Chin tucking.
   - Anticlockwise/backward rotation of the scapulae

Chronic stage is characterized by restriction of ROM in capsular pattern and pain at the end of range of motion with leathery end feel. Pain experienced during activities, but not at rest.

Aim

- Increase the extensibility of the shortened joint capsule and restore pain free full ROM.
- Strengthen the muscle
- Return to activities
- Prevent recurrence.

Means

- *Deep heating modalities* such as ultrasound, SWD and MWD can improve extensibility of collagen fibers of the joint capsule. But US is better.

- *Mobilization*

a. *Lateral distraction (Fig. 4.1)*

Starting position: Supine lying arm by the side with elbow flexed and forearm supported over the patient's abdomen.

Physiotherapist holds the lower end of arm by one hand and applies laterally directed pressure by the other hand placing it as high as possible in the axilla.

b. *Inferior gliding (Fig. 4.2)*

Starting position: Supine lying arm by the side

Physiotherapist standing towards the foot end of the bed grasps around the lower end of arm by one hand and above the wrist by the other hand. Pull it down to apply longitudinal caudal gliding.

Alternately physiotherapist standing towards the head end of the bed applies caudal gliding over the head of humerus, placing the thumbs or heel of the hand just lateral to the acromion (Fig. 4.3).

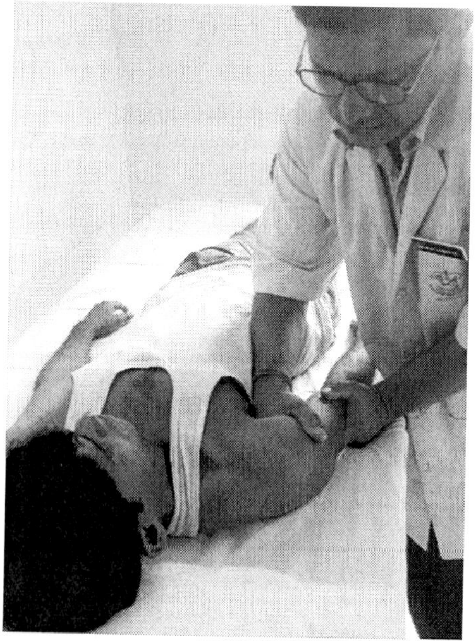

Fig. 4.1: Lateral distraction of humeral head over glenoid fossa

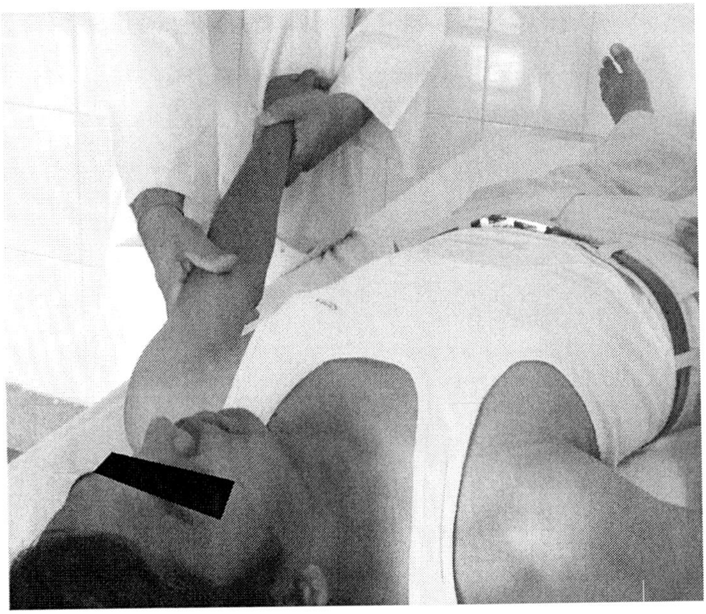

Fig. 4.2: Inferior/caudal glide of head of humerus

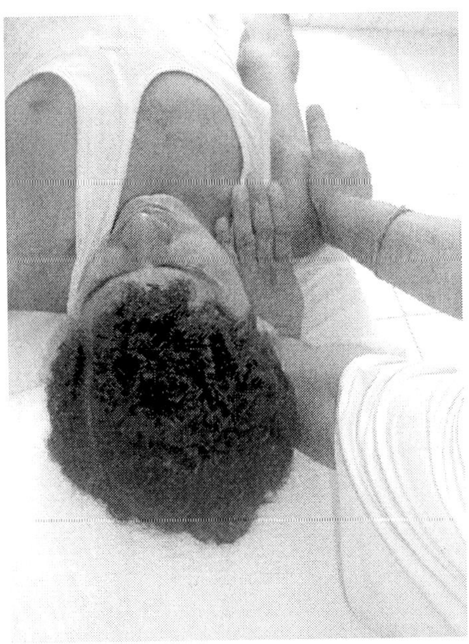

Fig. 4.3: Alternate method of inferior/caudal glide

Caudal gliding can be applied with the arm abducted, flexed or elevated position (Fig. 4.4) in supine or prone position.

c. Mobilization for shoulder external rotation, posterior-anterior gliding to stretch anterior joint capsule (Fig. 4.5).

   Starting position: Prone lying with arm abducted and laterally rotated with elbow flexed and forearm rested.

   Physiotherapist standing by the side applies posterior to anteriorly directed pressure over the head of humerus.

   Alternately patient in supine, physiotherapist in standing facing towards the patient grasps the upper end of humerus by both hands with fingers on the front and thumbs on the posterior aspect, mobilizes the head anterior to posteriorly by the fingers for internal rotation and posterior to anteriorly by the thumbs for external rotation (Fig. 4.9).

d. Mobilization for shoulder abduction, superior to inferior gliding to stretch inferior joint capsule (Fig. 4.6).

   Starting position: Supine lying with arm abducted

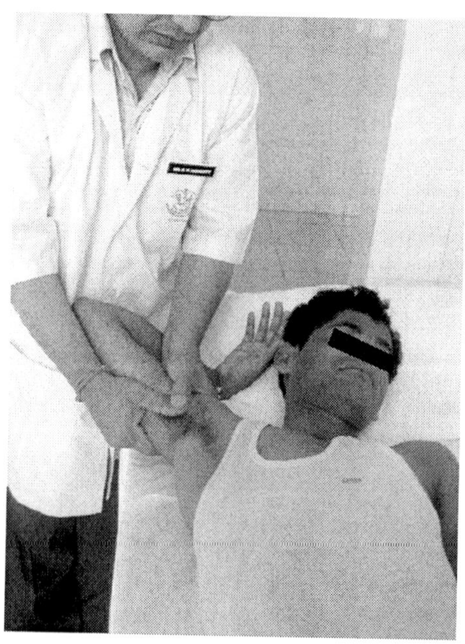

Fig. 4.4: End range caudal glide to improve elevation

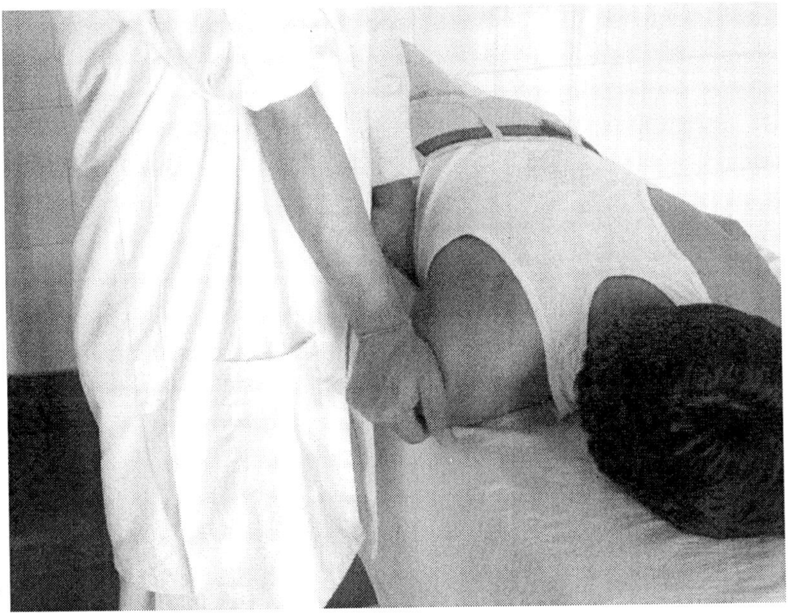

Fig. 4.5: PA glide to improve external rotation and extension range

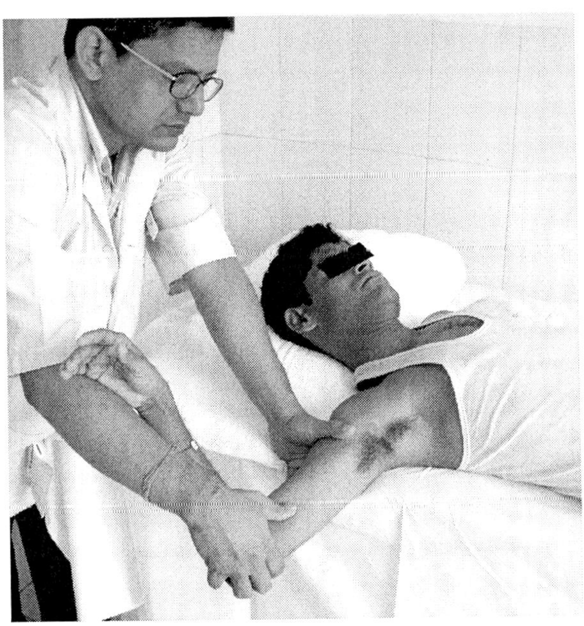

Fig. 4.6: Superior to inferior (caudal) glide to improve abduction range

Physiotherapist standing at the head end of the patient holds the lower end of arm and supports the forearm by one hand superior to inferiorly directed pressure is applied over the head of humerus.

Mobilization can be applied in sitting position with arm abducted (Fig. 4.7).

e. Mobilisation for shoulder internal rotation, anterior to posterior gliding to stretch posterior joint capsule (Fig. 4.8).

Starting position: supine lying arm by the side with elbow flexed and forearm supported over the patient's abdomen.

Physiotherapist holds the lower end of arm by one hand and anterior to posteriorly directed pressure is applied over the head of humerus by the thenar eminence of other hand.

Alternately, physiotherapist sits by the side of the patient with the thumbs on the posterior aspect of head of humerus and fingers of one hand spread over the clavicular region and those of other hand over the deltoid, mobilizes the head anterior to posteriorly by the fingers for internal rotation and posterior to anteriorly by the thumbs for external rotation (Fig. 4.9).

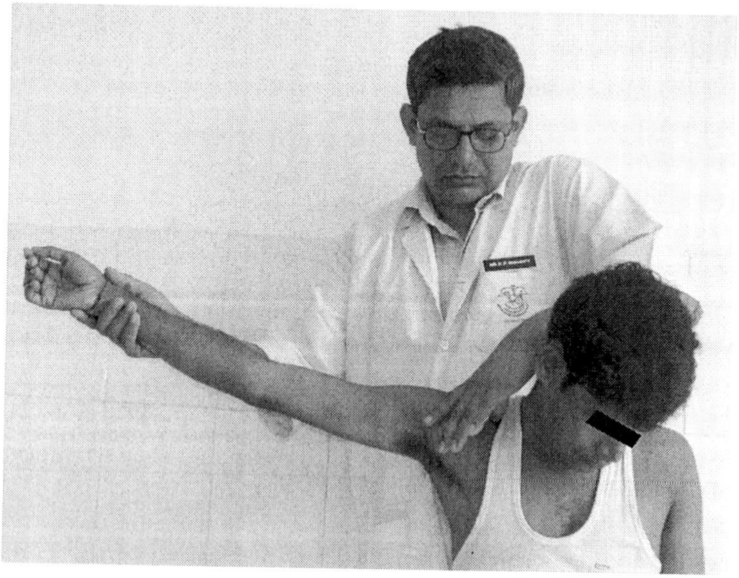

Fig. 4.7: Superior to inferior (caudal) glide in sitting to improve abduction range

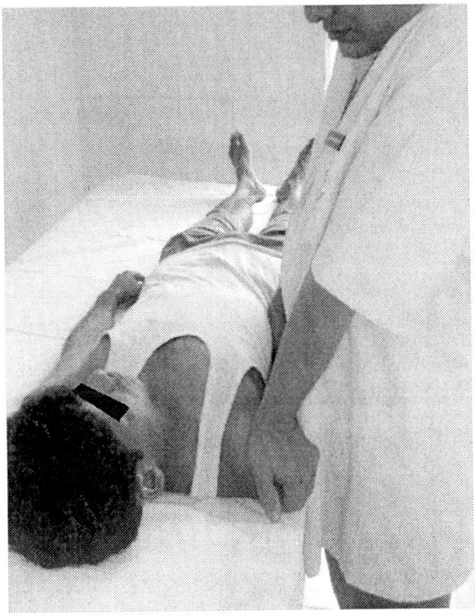

Fig. 4.8: Anterior to posterior glide to improve internal rotation and flexion range

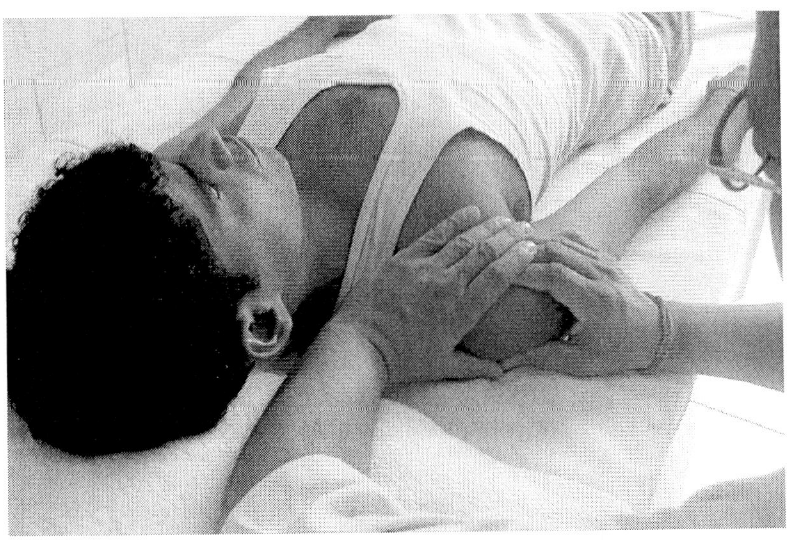

Fig. 4.9: AP/PA gliding of head of humerus over glenoid cavity

In supine lying position with the arm flexed to about 90°, therapist applies laterally distracted force by one hand and anterior to posteriorly directed force through the bent elbow by the other hand reinforced by the chin to stretch the posterior structures to improve the internal rotation range (Fig. 4.10). Scouring can be done for further benefits.

f. *Mobilization for shoulder elevation*

Starting position: Supine lying with arm behind the head

Physiotherapist standing at the head end of the patient holds the lower end of arm by one hand and applies cephalic to caudal gliding by the other hand (Fig. 4.4).

Alternately, in prone with hand behind head with one hand therapist support the bent elbow and with other hand applies caudal glide to stretch inferior capsule for abduction or anterior glide to stretch anterior capsule for external rotation range.

Automobilization exercises to do at home.

- In standing position with the affected arm abducted to 90°, elbow flexed to 90° and forearm supported over the wall, try to rotate the trunk towards opposite side to

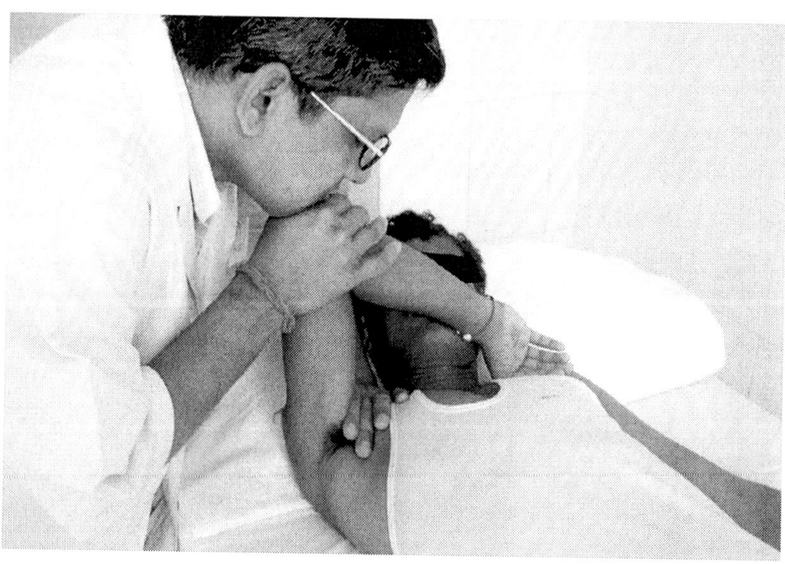

Fig. 4.10: Scouring to stretch posterior capsule to improve shoulder internal rotation range

experience stretching type of discomfort on the front of the shoulder due to stretching of anterior joint capsule (Fig. 4.11).

- Hold a stick by both the hands behind the head and move it backward.
- Keeping hand on back of head press the elbow backwards.
- In standing position with the affected arm flexed to 90° supported on the wall, turn the trunk towards the wall to experience stretching type of discomfort on the back of the shoulder due to stretching of posterior joint capsule (Fig. 4.12).
- Hold a small towel, one end by sound hand behind the neck and other end by involved hand behind the lower back and move it as if cleaning the back (Fig. 4.13) and vice-versa.

g. Weight and pulley exercises can be done for joint mobilization and strengthening of muscles. Theraband exercises are also useful.

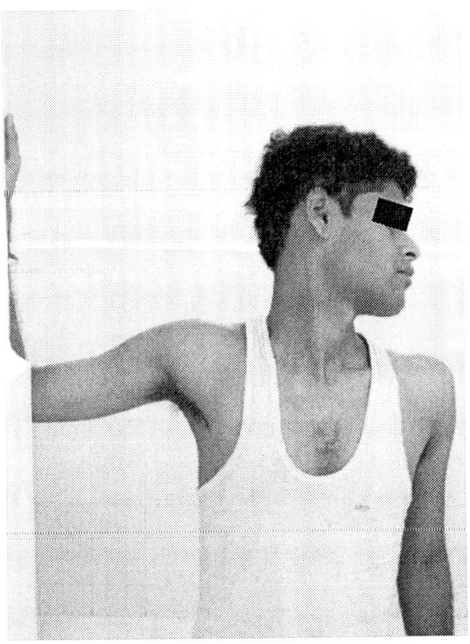

Fig. 4.11: Auto stretching of anterior shoulder capsule to improve external rotation

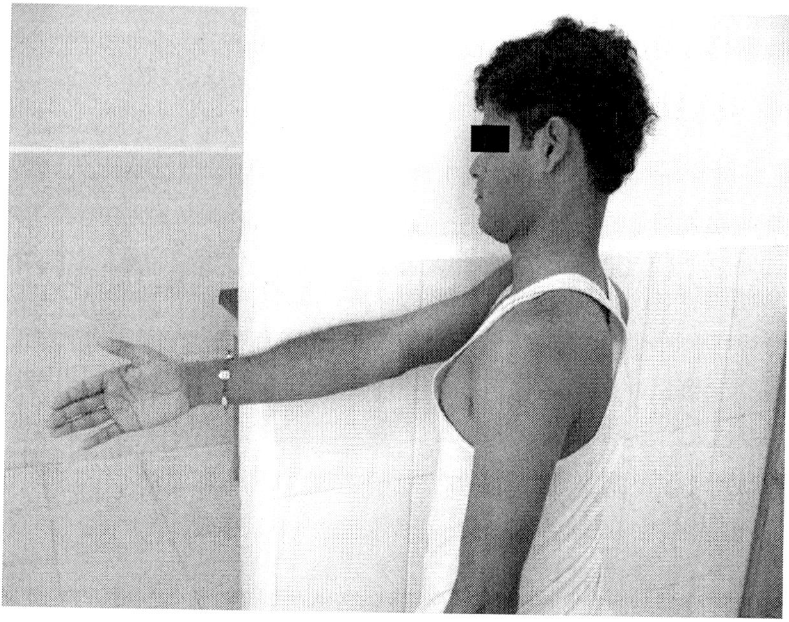

Fig. 4.12: Auto stretching of posterior shoulder capsule to improve internal rotation range

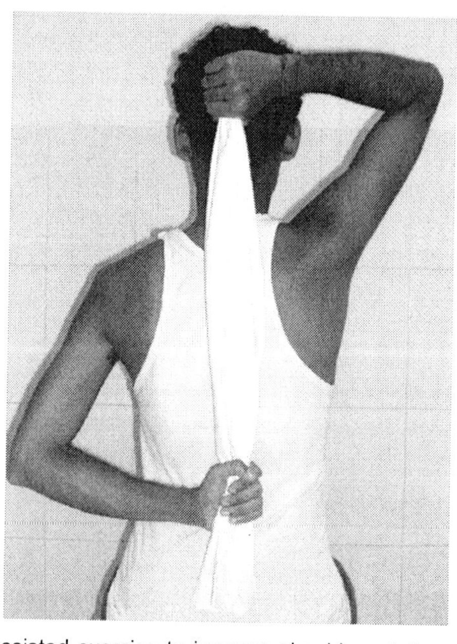

Fig. 4.13: Auto-assisted exercise to improve shoulder rotations range of motion

h. *Cyriax's capsular stretching in supine (Fig. 4.14)*
Starting position: Supine lying arm elevated as far as possible with keeping the hand in front forehead or under the head.

Physiotherapist stands facing towards the patient keeps one hand over the lower sternum to stabilize the thorax and presses the patient's elbow towards the couch to increase elevation. Hold it for some time and relax, then repeat the same with increase pressure. Progressively rotation can be added cautiously.

i Mulligan's method of mobilization to improve shoulder range internal rotation range (Fig. 4.15):

Starting position: sitting on a stool or standing holding the wrist of the affected hand by the sound hand behind the back and lifts it as high as possible.

Physiotherapist stands by the side facing towards the patient, keeps the thumb web space of one hand over the bent elbow while stabilizing the scapula with the other hand by applying upward and inwardly directed force. For the right shoulder glide the head of the humerus down in

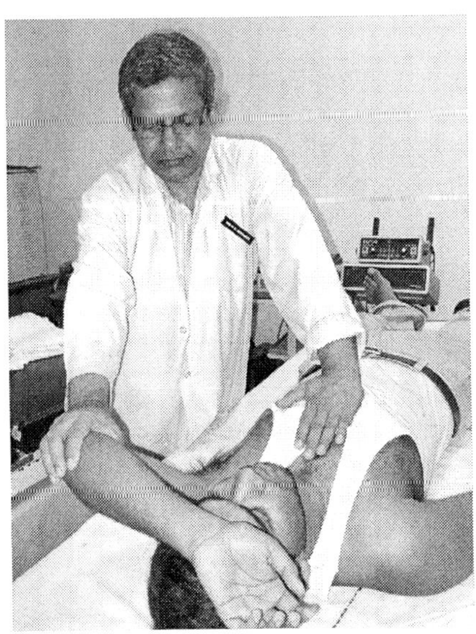

Fig. 4.14: Cyriax's capsular stretching

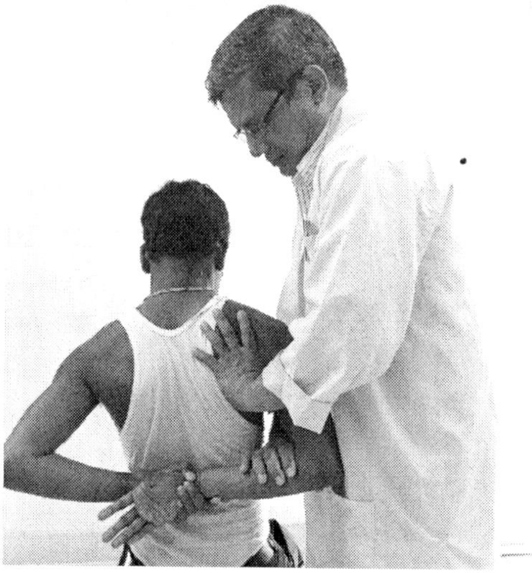

Fig. 4.15: Mulligan's mobilization to improve shoulder internal rotation range

the glenoid fossa by applying downwardly directed force over the bent elbow by the right hand and internally rotate the arm. The left hand which stabilizes the scapula also distracts the humeral head laterally and adduct patient's arm by your abdomen.

j. Mulligan's method of mobilization with movement for abduction-elevation:

Starting position: Sitting on a stool or standing

Physiotherapist stands by the side, for right shoulder place the right hand over the scapula and thenar eminence of left hand over the front of the head of humerus. Apply posteriorly directed force over the head while patient abducts and elevates the arm by the side. Mobilization is given at right angles, so that painless movement will take place. Then repeat it under load by giving weight to lift.

It can be done by using belt. Therapist stands behind the patient with the belt placed over the patient's shoulder and around your hips to apply posterior glide.

Mulligan's mobilization with movements for shoulder rotation is given in supine lying with arm flexed to 90° and elbow flexed and lateral rotation is performed while distraction applied by the belt.

- *Strengthening to* correct the muscle imbalance between rotator cuff vs. deltoid and trapizeus vs. serratus anterior
- Posture should be taken care of to prevent recurrence. Chin tucking, bilateral arm elevation and backward rotation of both scapulae help to correct the kyphotic posture.

Bulgen et al. (1984) in a long-term prospective study divided 42 subjects into four groups intra-articular injection, mobilizations, ice therapy and control group. All subjects were taught pendular exercises 2–3 minutes every hour and pain medication, if required.

Mobilization group: Maitland's mobilizations three times weekly for 6 weeks.

Ice therapy group: Ice pack followed by PNF three times weekly for 6 weeks. Steroid group: Intra-articular/subacromial injection weekly for 3 weeks.

Non-treatment group: Pendular exercises and pain medication.

Follow-up period: Weekly for the first 6 weeks then monthly for a further 6 months.

Outcome measures were verbal reports of progress, passive ROM (goniometry), total flexion, total abduction, external rotation, glenohumeral flexion, internal rotation. Results show that at six weeks, i.e. the end of treatment the groups were significantly different at the 2% level in steroid group.

Guler-Uysal et al (2004) in his study of comparison of the early response to two methods of rehabilitation in adhesive capsulitis, two groups were taken. Sample size was 40 and 3-week intervention. Active stretching and pendulum movements were performed by both groups after each session.

Experimental group received Cyriax's deep transverse frictions and manipulation performed by same experienced physiotherapist (1 hour session three times weekly). Control group received hot packs and short wave diathermy, 1 hour session 5 times weekly.

Follow-up period was end of 1 and 2 weeks. Outcome measures were pain using VAS: Spontaneous pain, night pain,

pain with motion, passive ROM (goniometry): Flexion, abduction, internal rotation, external rotation and recovery rate.

Result was 19 patients in the Cyriax group (95%) and 13 patients in the control group (65%) reached sufficient ROM at the end of the second week ($p < 0.05$). The improvement in shoulder flexion, inner and outer rotation values and the decrease in pain with motion were significantly better in the Cyriax group after the first week of treatment.

The Cyriax method requires fewer hospital visits, enabling the patients to proceed in their daily and professional activities. No special equipment is needed for the method but only an experienced health professional competent in the technique. The manipulation used during the Cyriax approach is mild and does not require anesthesia. It provides a health-care advantage during the active treatment period and this is of major importance for both the patient and the overloaded physical therapy clinics of referral hospitals.

Nicholson (1985) in his study on the Effects of Passive Joint Mobilization on Pain and Hypomobility associated with adhesive capsulitis of the Shoulder. Twenty subjects with adhesive capsulitis were divided into two groups. 4-week intervention was given. Experimental group received gliding and distractive mobilization techniques and exercises, 2–3 weekly for 4 weeks. In the early sessions gliding and distractive mobilization techniques were performed with the joint near its neutral position, progressing in the later sessions to mobilization toward the end of the range of motion. During abduction, for instance, inferior glide of the humerus was performed with the shoulder in approximately 25' of abduction; subsequently progression to inferior glide at the individual's limit of abduction. Control group received exercises alone. Follow-up period was weekly for 4 weeks. During the treatment sessions, the control subjects performed active exercises in those ranges found to be restricted and additional resistive exercises if weaknesses were present. The controls were instructed to repeat the exercises three times per day independently.

Outcome measures were pain questionnaire, ROM (goniometry): Active internal rotation, Active external rotation active abduction, passive abduction. Pain questionnaires were answered and isolated glenohumeral mobility measurements were taken initially and at weekly intervals during the 4 weeks of treatment. With the exception of internal rotation in the control group, all motions increased significantly from baseline in both groups. Passive abduction improved significantly more in the mobilization group than in the control group. Pain scores decreased more in the mobilization group; however, the difference between the groups was not significant. The results suggest that joint mobilization and exercises are clinically effective in the treatment of painfully stiff shoulders.

Moritz stated that, from a biomechanical viewpoint, passive mobilization techniques are preferred over conventional passive range of motion exercises, especially in conditions of reduced load tolerance of the joint structures. Because of the leverage effect of the conventional passive exercises, a compression force is produced on the articular surfaces and a stretching of the periarticular structures occur which is much greater than the external force applied. **Lundberg** found a significant degree of osteoporosis associated with frozen shoulder which indicates that leverage or compression should be minimized during the treatment.

Vermeulen et al (2000) in his case report describes the use of end-range mobilization techniques in the management of patients with adhesive capsulitis. Four men and three women with adhesive capsulitis of the glenohumeral joint were treated with end-range mobilization techniques, twice a week for 3 months. Indexes of pain, joint mobility, and function were measured by the same observer before treatment, after 3 months of treatment, and at the time of a 9-month follow-up. In addition, arthrographic assessment of joint capacity, i.e., the amount of fluid the joint can contain and measurement of range of motion of glenohumeral abduction on a plain radiograph were conducted initially and after 3 months of treatment.

Intervention using end-range mobilization techniques as described by Maitland started after the radiological assessment and was given twice a week for 30 minutes. Intervention started with a few minutes of warm up consisting of rhythmic mid-range mobilizations with the patient in a supine position. After 10 to 15 repetitions of intensive mobilization techniques in this end-range position, the direction of mobilization was altered by varying the plane of elevation or by varying the degree of rotation. In addition, as an alternative to varying the direction of mobilization, other movements such as gliding techniques and distraction in that joint position were used. In each direction of mobilization, 10 to 15 repetitions were performed, and the mobilization grade (3 or 4) and the duration of prolonged stress varied according to the patient's tolerance.

Outcomes: After 3 months of treatment, there were increases in active range of motion. Mean abduction, flexion in the sagittal, and mean lateral rotation increased. There were also increases in passive range of motion .The mean capacity of the glenohumeral joint capsule increased from 10 cc to 15 cc.

Vermeulen et al (2006) in his study compared the effectiveness of high-grade mobilization techniques (HGMT) with that of low-grade mobilization techniques (LGMT) in subjects with adhesive capsulitis of the shoulder. In this study, 100 subjects with unilateral adhesive capsulitis were taken. Low-grade mobilization group got Maitland grade I and II joint mobilization and high grade mobilization group got Maitland grade III and IV joint mobilization. Outcome measures were active and passive ROM by goniometry for abduction, forward flexion, external rotation, shoulder rating questionnaire (SRQ), shoulder disability questionnaire (SDQ), pain using VAS: Pain at rest, pain during movement, pain during the night measured.

In both groups, subjects were treated twice per week for 30 minutes for a maximum of 12 weeks and were encouraged to attend all treatment sessions. If the therapist noticed a normal ROM relative to the unaffected side, then reducing the frequency to once per week and stopping the treatment were permitted, provided that each subject had a minimal duration of exposure to the therapy of at least 6 weeks. In both groups, subjects did not receive a home exercise program but were advised to use the affected shoulder in daily activities whenever possible.

In both the groups, every session started with a 5-minute assessment of the ROM by performing all 3 physiologic movements of the glenohumeral joint passively with the subject in the supine position. At each position of the shoulder, the end-feel of the movement was assessed in order to apply the mobilization techniques into the stiffness zone (HGMT group) or within the pain-free zone (LGMT group). If the glenohumeral joint ROM increased during treatment, then mobilization techniques were performed at greater elevation and abduction angles. In these new positions, the changed position of the humeral head and glenoid required an individual adjustment of the direction of the accessory movements in accordance with the concave-convex rules stated by Kaltenborn.

Overall, subjects in both groups improved over 12 months. Statistically significant greater change scores were found in the HGMT group for passive abduction (at the time points 3 and 12 months), and for active and passive external rotation (at 12 months). A statistically significant difference in trend between both groups over the total follow-up period of 12 months was found for passive external rotation, SRQ, and SDQ with greater change scores in the HGMT group.

Jing-lan Yang et al (2007) in his study Mobilization Techniques in Subjects with Frozen Shoulder Syndrome—Randomized Multiple Treatment Trial—there were 3 groups—end-range mobilization (ERM), mid-range mobilization (MRM), and mobilization with movement (MWM)—in the management of subjects with frozen shoulder syndrome (FSS). 28 subjects with frozen shoulder syndrome were recruited. The duration of each treatment was 3 weeks, for a total of 12 weeks. Outcome measures included the functional score and shoulder kinematics.

Results: Overall, subjects in both groups improved over the 12 weeks. Statistically significant improvements were found in

ERM and MWM. Additionally, MWM corrected scapulohumeral rhythm significantly better than ERM did.

Conclusion: In subjects with frozen shoulder syndrome, ERM and MWM were more effective than MRM in increasing mobility and functional ability.

Andrea Johnson et al (2007) in his study compared the effect of anterior versus posterior glide joint mobilization on external rotation range of motion in patients with shoulder adhesive capsulitis: Twenty consecutive subjects with a primary diagnosis of shoulder adhesive capsulitis and exhibiting a specific external rotation ROM deficit were randomly assigned to 1 of 2 treatment groups. All subjects received 6 therapy sessions consisting of application of therapeutic ultrasound, joint mobilization and upper-body ergometer exercise.

Ultrasound was administered to the anterior capsule of those in the anterior glide joint mobilization group and to the posterior capsule of those in the posterior glide joint mobilization group, with the intent to provide the target tissue which is deemed adequate to alter the viscoelastic properties of connective tissue. In general, most posterior capsules were treated using 1-MHz ultrasound because it was determined that the capsule was 2 to 5 cm deep and most anterior capsules were treated with 3 MHz, as the capsule was determined to be 0.5 to 2 cm deep (**Draper DO et al**).

Joint mobilizations were followed the ultrasound treatment as soon as the subject could be positioned appropriately. To minimize joint compression and possible periarticular soft tissue damage, lateral traction of the glenohumeral joint was performed before and during the mobilization procedures.

The joint mobilization procedures used in this study were stretch mobilizations, which loaded the restricting tissue at a slow rate and maintained a low load over a prolonged period at the end of the available abduction and/or external rotation ROM with a linear, gliding movement produced by bone translation. These were Kaltenborn grade III mobilizations, which apply force after the slack of the joint has been taken up, to stretch tissues crossing the joint. The end range position of the mobilization was held for at least 1 minute. No oscillatory motions were performed. Each stretch mobilization was repeated so that a total of 15 minutes of sustained stretch was performed at each treatment session.

A significant difference between groups (P = .001) was present by the third treatment. The individuals in the anterior mobilization group had a mean improvement in external rotation ROM of 3.0° whereas the individuals in the posterior mobilization group had a mean improvement of 31.3°.

James Camarinos et al (2009) Effectiveness of Manual Physical Therapy for Painful Shoulder Conditions – Systematic Review: The purpose of this systematic review was to identify the effectiveness of manual therapy to the glenohumeral joint across all painful shoulder conditions. A search of MEDLINE, CINAHL, Web of Science, and Cochrane Central Register of Randomized Controlled Trials for articles dated **1996 to June 2009** was performed. Inclusion for review were manual therapy performed to the glenohumeral joint only; non-surgical painful shoulder disorders; subjects 18–80 years; and outcomes of range of motion, pain, function, and/or quality of life. Quality assessment was performed using the PEDro scale with subsequent data extraction. Seventeen related articles were found with seven fitting the inclusion criteria. The average PEDro score was 7.86, meeting the cut off score for high quality. Significant heterogeneity in outcome measures prohibited meta-analysis. Five studies demonstrated benefits utilizing manual therapy for mobility, and four demonstrated a trend towards decreasing pain values. Functional outcomes and quality-of-life measures varied greatly among all studies. Manual therapy appears to increase either active or passive mobility of the shoulder. A trend was found favoring manual therapy for decreasing pain, but the effect on function and quality of life remains inconclusive. Future research utilizing consistent outcome measurements is necessary.

BIBLIOGRAPHY

1. Andua Johnson, et al. The effect of anterior versus posterior glide joint mobilisation on external rotation Raye of motion in patient with shoulder adhesive capsulitis, 2007.
2. Bulgen, et al. Frozen shoulder, a long term prospective study 1984.
3. Cyriax J: Textbook of orthopaedic medicine, vol 1: diagosis of soft tissue lesions, edn 8, London Bailliere - Tindall.
4. Cyriax J: Textbook of orthopaedic medicine, vol 2, edn 11, London, 1984, Bailliere - Tindall 1982.
5. Donatelli RA: physical therapy of the shoulder, 2nd edition; Churchill Livingstone 1991.
6. Fusun guler – vysal et al. Compansion of the cally response to 2 methods of rehabilitation in adhesive capsulitis 2002.
7. Hertling D, Kessler RM: Management of common musculoskeletal disorders, edn 2. Philadelphia, Lippincott 1990.
8. James Camarinos, et al. Effectiveness of manual physical therapy for painful shoulder condition. A Systemic Review, 2009.
9. Jinglar Yang, et al. Mobilisation technique is subject with frozen shoulder syndrome. Randomized multiple treatment trial 2007.
10. Kisner C, Colby LA: Therapeutic exercise: foundations and techniques, edn 2, Philadelphia, FA Davis 1990.
11. Maitland GO: Treatment of the glenohumeral joint by passive movement. Physiotherapy 1983;69:3-7.
12. Neviaser JS: Adhesive capsulitis of the shoulder. J Bone Joint Surg 1945;27:211-22.
13. Neviaser JS: Adhesive capsulitis of the siff and painful shoulder. Orthop Clin North Am 1980;11:327-33.
14. Nicholson GG: The effects of passive joint mobilizataion on pain and hypomobility associated with adhesive capsulitis of the shoulder. Orthop Sports Phys Ther 1985;6:238-46.
15. Nicholson, et al. Effect of passive joint mobilisation on pain and hypomobility associated with adhesive capsulitis of shoulder 1985.
16. Reevs B: The natural history of the frozen shoulder syndrome, Scand J Rheumatol 1975;4:193-6.
17. Vermeuler, et al. Companion of high grade and low grade mobilisation in mangement of adhesive capsulitis of shoulder. Randomized Controlled Trial, 2006.
18. Vermulon, et al. Endrange mobilisation technique in adhesive capsulitis of shoulder joint a multiple subject case report 2000.
19. Wadsworth CT: Frozen shoulder, Phys Ther 1986;66(12): 1878-83.

Chapter 5

Thoracic Outlet Syndrome

Thoracic outlet syndrome (TOS) sometimes referred as thoracic inlet syndrome (TIS) is one of the commonly overlooked conditions. Patient reporting with the complaint of upper extremity pain is often diagnosed as cervical spondylosis or PID. The thoracic outlet syndrome refers to a series of neurovascular compression in the shoulder region. Subclavian vessels and/or lower trunk or medial cord of brachial plexus get compressed at either sternocostovertebral space, scalene triangle, costoclavicular space or coracopectoral space. The boundary of thoracic outlet is formed by scalenus anticus anteriorly, scalenus medius posteriorly, clavicle superiorly and first rib inferiorly (Fig. 5.1). The brachial plexus travels between the scalenus anticus and medius (scalene triangle) into the supraclavicular region, where the ventral primary rami unite to form the superior, middle and inferior trunks. Ventral rami of C8 and T1 unite to form inferior trunk, which enters the axilla by crossing between clavicle and first rib (costoclavicular space). After leaving the costoclavicular space the nerve passes infraclavicularly underneath pectoralis minor (coracopectoral space). Symptoms related to compression of brachial plexus such as pain, paresthesia, weakness, etc. are found in about 90% of all TOS, whereas symptoms related to compression of vessels such as edema, heaviness, weakness and Raynaud's phenomenon (cyanosed, blanching and erythema), etc. are found in about 10% of all TOS.

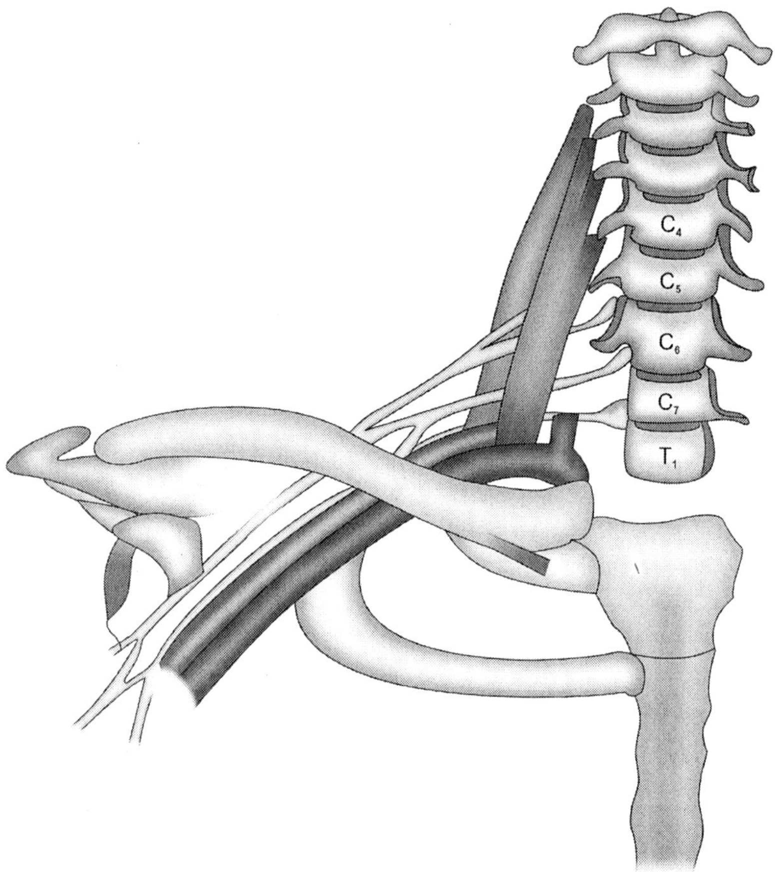

Fig. 5.1: Boundary of thoracic outlets

ETIOLOGY

Three categories of risk factors in the development of TOS are:

1. Congenital-structural anomaly
2. Traumatic structural alterations in the size of thoracic outlet
3. Postural alterations in the size of thoracic outlet

Congenital Factors

Cervical rib, which articulates with the transverse process of seventh cervical vertebra, is present in 1% of the population and only 10% of all with cervical ribs develop symptoms of TOS. It extends into the neck where its anterior end may either be free or attachéd to the first rib or sternum.

Long transverse process of seventh cervical vertebra may give rise to TOS.

Sometimes anomalous fibrous band originate either from the end of C7 transverse process or from the end of a short cervical rib and inserts on the first thoracic rib, which may cause as much trouble as bony rib though, cannot be detected radiographically.

Abnormal scalene muscle development, which is often associated with anomalous fibromuscular bands within these muscles, may entrap upper trunk of brachial plexus.

Normally such structural anomaly may cause little or no trouble. They represent a risk factor in the development of TOS following trauma or postural alteration.

Traumatic Factors

Malunited fracture clavicle: The extra callus forms at the fracture site significantly diminishes the space between clavicle and first rib.

Whiplash tears of scalene muscle: Increased scalene muscle tone elevates the first rib and reduces thoracic outlet dimension. Reflex muscle spasm of scalene compresses the portion of the plexus that travels within the intrascalene space. The fibrosed scar contracture following tear of the scalene muscle due to whiplash injury may also compress the portion of the plexus passing through it.

Postural Factors

Middle aged women are more affected than men with 3:1 ratio. The upper margin of the sternum is in level with lower part of the second dorsal vertebra in males and lower part of the third dorsal vertebra in females. In the female, the medial third of clavicle is lower than that in the male and thereby diminishes the space between clavicle and first rib.

Females with large breasts attaching to the pectoralis major muscle exert a downward pull over the sternal half of the clavicle further reducing the thoracic outlet dimension.

Normally with elevation of arm, clavicle rotates backward reducing the costoclavicular space. Elevation of first rib during deep inspiration, downward depression of clavicle during carrying heavy weights, backward and downward movement of clavicle during retraction of shoulders also narrowed the costoclavicular space.

Upper trapezius elevates the clavicle and prevents shoulder girdle from sagging down on the chest. Drooping shoulder, which is associated with pregnancy, stooping posture, head forward posture, negative psychological state, etc. reduces the thoracic outlet dimension. Wearing heavy overcoat, carrying heavy weight by hand, simply holding the arm in dependent position for any length of time, etc. also precipitate or predispose TOS.

The extraordinary mobility of the shoulder requires neurovascular structures to change its direction by as much as 180°. The coracoid process and the pectoralis minor act as a fulcrum for the change in direction and present one final potential site of compression before the neurovascular structures enter the axilla. Such incidences are seen in athletes, who frequently assume shoulder hyperabduction, e.g. swimming, serving and throwing, etc.

Pancoast tumor, also known as pulmonary superior sulcus tumor, present at sternocostovertebral space compresses the inferior trunk of brachial plexus, formed by C8 and T1 roots.

CLINICAL FEATURES

About 90% of all TOS show neurological signs and symptoms due to compression of medial cord, branch of lower trunk of brachial plexus (C8 and T1). Compression of ulnar nerve and the medial cutaneous nerve of forearm, branches of medial cord produces paresthesia may be accompanied by aching pain, often experienced over the medial aspect of forearm and hypothenar region of hand. The symptoms aggravate by carrying heavy weight or stooping posture. Patient often complains of clumsiness and weakness of fingers, which could be more due to sensory impairment than motor deficits. Motor deficits are not usually present in TOS. If present, there is weakness of grip strength or pinch strength, atrophy of intrinsic muscles of hand supplied by C8 and T1 roots in long-standing TOS.

In about 5–10% of all TOS vascular signs and symptoms include edema of hand, coldness, muscle ache and loss of strength on prolonged use. Compression of nerve trunk along with vascular insufficiency is second common involvement next to primary compression of lower trunk of brachial plexus, whereas isolated compression of subclavian vessels is rare and that of upper trunk of brachial plexus is uncommon.

Evaluation

Posture

Inspect from the front: Check the shoulder heights (depressed/ elevated), scapular protraction, orientation of clavicle, symmetry of chest wall, breathing pattern, upper extremity attitude, wasting, etc.

From the back, check the shoulder heights (depressed/ elevated), scapular retraction, wasting of girdle muscles, etc. From the sides, check head forward posture, thoracic kyphosis, increased upper cervical lordosis, etc.

Sensory Evaluation

Cutaneous sensation of upper extremity can be evaluated by pressure sensitive Semmes Weinstein monofilaments. These nylon filaments are calibrated so that when a specific amount of pressure is applied to the tip, it bends indicating that the filament's threshold has been reached. Twenty filaments ranging from 0.0045 to 447 g can be used to map out sensory threshold and compare it with the uninvolved side.

The cutaneous sensation of the involved side at both symptom provocating and relieving postures can also be compared.

Sympathetic Evaluation (Sweat Test)

Ninhydrin Sweat Test

A few drops of 1% Ninhydrin is added to soak the filter paper, and allowed to dry. The filter paper punches are transferred to the adhesive side of a piece of scotch tape by using a nontouch technique and then applied to the skin site to be tested and its corresponding normal site. The patient is asked to walk in the sun to induce thermal sweating and the sweat function is graded after half an hour.

1 = no color change
2 = first perceptible blue-purple color change
3 = color change in between 1 and 4
4 = intense blue purple color change.

Quinizarin Sweat Test

The areas to be tested are first thoroughly dried and then liberally dusted with Quinizarin powder. The patient is placed under a heat cradle and given a hot drink combined with acetylsalicylic acid. Areas of sweat production are clearly outlined as the powder turns black when exposed to moisture. In sympathetic lesions there will be a segmental loss of sweating corresponding to the distribution of the affected sympathetic fibers. This is a good test for the results of sympathetectomy section or injury to the peripheral nerves and for demonstrating and photographing denervated areas. It can show objectively areas of sympathetic denervation.

Motor Evaluation

Thorough upper extremity manual muscle testing should be done to establish the site and extent of nerve involvement. Usually intrinsic muscles of hand supplied by ulnar nerve (C8 and T1) are involved.

Measurement of Edema

Volumetric Measurement

a. *Direct method:* The patient's hand is submerged in a graduated transparent container, which is half-filled with water and the volume of water displaced is recorded. Both the hands should be measured and the difference between the two indicates the amount of edema in ml/cc.
b. *Indirect method:* The patient's hand is submerged in a container, which is filled with water and placed over another to collect the displaced water. The amount of water displaced is measured in ml/cc using a calibrated cylinder. Both the hands should be measured and the difference between the two indicates the amount of edema in ml/cc.

Circumferential Measurement

The girth of the forearm at different levels from a particular bony reference point, e.g. tip of radial styloid process or olecranon process is measured by using flexible measure tape. Both the extremities should be measured and the difference between the two is recorded.

Peripheral Pulsations

Brachial and radial pulses should be palpated for rate and volume in both the extremities and compared. Pulsation of the involved extremity at both symptom provocating and relieving postures should also be compared.

Examination of Supraclavicular Fossa

Percussion or firm pressure over supraclavicular fossa may produce pain or paresthesia because of irritation of nerve trunk near the site of compression.

Palpable fibrous or fibromuscular band may be present at this region.

Provocative Tests

Adson's test, costoclavicular maneuver, hyperabduction test, overhead exercise test, Allen's test/Wright's maneuver are various special tests used clinically for the diagnosis of TOS. Upper extremity tension test particularly for ulnar nerve becomes positive.

Investigations

X-ray: AP view of the cervical spine including the clavicle may show cervical rib or long C7 transverse process. It also demonstrates any irregularity of the clavicle or first rib.

Electro-diagnosis: The diagnosis of TOS is not made easy by elctro-physiological studies, but useful in excluding the common differential diagnostic problems of distal entrapment neuropathy and cervical radiculopathy. EMG and NCV for ulnar nerve sensory action potential as well as motor conduction at elbow are done to rule out ulnar nerve lesion at elbow. Characteristic electrodiagnostic changes include but are not limited to prolonged latency of the ulnar F-wave and reduced amplitude of ulnar sensory evoked amplitude.

MRI: Magnetic resonance imaging or myelogram of cervical spine helps to clarify the level of nerve compression.

Arteriograms/Venograms are invasive vascular study performed to detect site and extent of subclavian vessel obstruction/dilatation. It is indicated in cases of arterial insufficiency and in the presence of complete cervical rib, which compresses the subclavian artery resulting into post-stenotic aneurysm.

Doppler ultrasound and photoplethysmography is often used to monitor blood flow during the provocative maneuver instead of palpation of radial pulse. Both the instruments are non-invasive with better sensitivity to detect subtle change in blood flow, so often preferred over arteriogram.

DIAGNOSIS

Thoracic outlet syndrome remains a clinical diagnosis based almost entirely on the history and physical examination. There is no single ancillary test that is able to confirm the diagnosis of TOS. There is high incidence of false positive and false negative results of the provocative tests. More than 50% of normal asymptomatic people will obliterate radial pulse during the provocative tests and only 5–10% of all TOS cases have vascular involvement. Therefore, obliteration of radial pulse is not reliable and the test must be considered positive only when the original symptoms are reproduced.

MANAGEMENT

There is general agreement that the initial treatment of thoracic outlet syndrome should be conservative. The goals of management are to avoid precipitating postures and activities, correct postural abnormalities that might be contributing to neurovascular compression, activities modification, environmental modifications and to strengthen the scapular suspensory musculature to maintain the correct posture.

Symptomatic therapy for pain relief includes ultrasound, ice, moist heat, massage, etc. to relieve spasm of upper trapezius. TENS, IFT, electrical stimulation, etc. can also be used for pain relief.

Unsupported weight of upper extremity depresses the shoulder girdle compressing the neurovascular structures, demanding reflex contraction of scalene, sternocleidomastoid and upper trapezius to elevate the shoulder, which in turn compresses the upper plexus. So to avoid overcontraction of these muscles support the extremity passively, on the table top or arm rest of the chair or pillow while sitting and by the sound hand or put it inside the pocket while standing. One should sleep using three pillows, one supporting the head and neck in slight flexion and others support the shoulders with scapulae in abduction.

Women with pendulous breasts must use well-supportive brassiere with extra padding of the shoulder straps or only back straps without shoulder straps may be used.

Stretching of levator scapulae, scalene, pectoralis minor and pectoralis major muscles to restore their normal length is very important.

Mobilization of sternoclavicular joint, scapulothoracic joint, first and second rib articulations increases thoracic cage flexibility.

Strengthening of upper trapezius and serratus anterior to maintain normal posture is important.

Diaphragmatic breathing reduces activities of accessory inspiratory muscles such as scalene and sternocleidomastoid. Otherwise hypertrophy of these muscles may compress the neurovascular structures.

Gentle brachial plexus gliding exercises to maintain or restore free excursion of brachial plexus within the upper extremity is recommended. For median nerve abduction and external rotation of shoulder followed by elbow extension and supination, wrist and finger extension and finally neck side flexion to the opposite side may be added gradually with little discomfort but no pain. For ulnar nerve abduction and external rotation of shoulder followed by elbow flexion and supination, wrist and finger extension and finally neck side flexion to the opposite side may be added gradually with little discomfort but no pain.

Weight reduction, relaxation, avoidance of wearing heavy overcoat, carrying heavy weight by hand, etc. are useful.

Surgical treatment may be considered when the conservative treatment fails and there is a progressing neurological deficit, acute vascular insufficiency or incapacitating pain. The surgical management is directed at the specific pathology that is present and the procedures include first rib resection through transaxillary approach, scalenectomy with or without rib resection through supraclavicular approach, severing of pectoralis minor muscle, trisection of subclavius muscle above the coracoid ligament, etc. Postoperative therapy includes maintenance or restoration of full range of motion, flexibility, strength, posture, neural gliding, etc.

BIBLIOGRAPHY

1. Donatelli RA: Physical therapy of the shoulder, 2nd edition; Churchill Livingstone 1991.
2. Elvey R: Brachial plexus tension tests and the pathoanatomical origin of arm pain. In: Glascon E, et al. (Editors) Aspects of manipulative therapy, edn 2, New York, 1985, Churchill Livingstone.
3. Hawkes C: Neurosurgical considerations in thoracic outlet syndrome. Clin Orthop 1980;207:24.
4. Hoffman J: Electrodiagnostic techniques for and conservative treatment of thoracic outlet syndrome. Clin Orthop 1986;207:21.
5. Kisner C, Colby LA: Therapeutic exercise: foundations and techniques, edn 2. Philadelphia, FA Davis 1990.
6. Smith KF: The thoracic outlet syndrome: A protocol of treatment. J Orthop Sports Phys Ther 1979;1(2):89-97.

Chapter

6

Fractures and Dislocations

FRACTURE OF CLAVICLE

It is one of the commonest injuries of upper extremity. Fracture occurs at the middle third of the bone from fall on outstretched hand or fall on the shoulder. The lateral segment is displaced forwards and downwards by the weight of the limb, while the medial segment is displaced upwards by the pull of sternocleidomastoid muscle. There is often overlapping giving rise to chest asymmetry, i.e. affected side chest becomes short. The sharp edge of fracture segment sometimes projects forward damaging the overlying skin. Rarely it may be displaced backwards and endanger the subclavian vessels. The fracture is clinically united within 3–4 weeks and functional recovery is complete within about 2–3 months. Accurate reduction is neither possible nor essential.

Indication of surgery:
- Compound #
- Associated NV compromise
- Established nonunion

Malunited thickened fracture site reduces the thoracic outlet dimension giving rise to thoracic outlet syndrome (TOS).

Management

Overlapping of fracture ends can be corrected by retracting the shoulders and applying figure of 8 bandages in-between the shoulders. Downward displacement is corrected by triangular sling supporting the elbow and forearm, tied over the opposite shoulder. Immobilization is given for 4–6 weeks, during which fingers, wrist; forearm and elbow movements are encouraged. It takes 3 months for functional recovery to take place. Avoid overhead activity as it rotates clavicle backward, carrying weight by hand and lying on affected side shoulder up to 3 months of fracture. After removal of immobilization, apply moist heat to relax the muscles around the shoulder followed by pendular exercises. Shoulder rotation can be done.

Surgery is indicated in a very few cases where sharp fracture edge of bone endangers the underlying vessels or overlying skin. Flexible intramedullary nail fixation or clavicular plate fixation is done. Post-operatively sling support is given for about 6 weeks. Pin is removed after 3 months. Non-union may occur by the internal fixation, which strips its blood supply.

Complications:
- Subclavian artery injury by # beak
- Brachial plexus injury especially medial cord nerve symptoms
- Pneumothorax
- Nonunion (in lateral 1/3rd clavicle #)

FRACTURE OF GREATER TUBEROSITY

It can occur in adults at any age but common in elderly. There are two types of fracture greater tuberosity:
1. Contusion occurs due to direct blow. It occurs due to fall on the tip of the shoulder. May be associated with fracture neck of humerus or dislocation of the shoulder. Comminuted fragments are usually undisplaced by the periosteum.
2. Avulsion occurs due to forceful adduction during strong contraction of abductors. The greater tuberosity from the insertion site of rotator cuff is pulled off. It is almost always displaced.

From management point of view, it is important to detect whether the fracture is displaced or undisplaced.

Undisplaced fractures are managed like soft tissue injury. A sling support for 1–2 weeks is applied. Immediately active fingers, wrist, forearm and elbow movements are encouraged. After a few days once the acute responses are subsided, active assisted movements of the shoulder can be started. Restoration of movements and muscle strength will be regained within a few weeks and patient returns to activities.

Displaced fractures with minimal displacement due to intact capsule and periosteum fibers are managed by sling support for 3 weeks.

Completely displaced large fracture segments are managed by surgical fixation with consensus screws whereas small segments can be fixed by intraosseus suture.

FRACTURE OF SURGICAL NECK OF HUMERUS

Fracture of surgical neck of humerus occurs mostly in elderly women because of osteoporosis.

Mode of injury: Fall on outstretched hand or on elbow.

Following fracture, there is displacement, the degree of displacement varies from mild to severe. Strong pull of the rotator cuff tilts the head in the direction of abduction, so the shaft appears adducted in relation to the head. Strong pull of the deltoid abducts shaft of humerus in relation to the head. In case of unstable fracture, there is chance of displacement and redisplacement.

Stable fractures are either impacted or undisplaced. Distal fracture segment pierces into proximal segment and appears as a single segment. In stable fracture, considerable amount of shoulder movements occur with little discomfort.

Diagnosis

- Elderly women
- H/o fall on outstretched hand or elbow
- Ecchymosis on lateral aspect of arm, first red and then blue
  Prolong immobilization following reduction in elderly

women gives rise to stiffness of shoulder joint, so should be avoided.

Aim

- Early mobilization
- Perfect reduction is difficult except surgery, but small proximal segment makes it difficult to fix by surgical procedure.
- With the displacement, good functional recovery is possible, So conservative management is preferred.

Management

Stable Fracture

It is left like that or at best 3 weeks of sling support can be given. One can remove the sling to do gravity assisted positional exercises with little discomfort, but no pain as the initial acuteness subsides. No activity should be done.

Unstable Fracture

Elderly Persons

2-3 weeks sling support. In some cases 3-4 weeks abduction splint immobilization.

After 3 weeks, as the fracture site is glued and becomes stable enough, active assisted movement with little discomfort should be practiced. Positional movements should be encouraged. Forward leaning produces shoulder flexion, sideway leaning produces abduction.

Young Persons

Closed manipulative reduction under anesthesia followed by shoulder spica immobilization with the shoulder in abducted position for 4 weeks.

Open reduction and internal fixation is rarely done as the small proximal fracture segment is difficult to fix. But in some may be done by intramedullary nail or screw plate fixation.

Postoperative immobilization depends on the degree of stability achieved by operation. In case of stable fixation, the arm is held in a roller towel abduction sling for a few days, following which active exercises are started.

Physiotherapy during immobilization aims at restoration of function by preventing complications. Static biceps and triceps contractions compress the fracture site and stimulate osteogenesis.

Postimmobilization physiotherapy:

1. Hot pack to relax muscles around the shoulder joint.
2. Pendular exercises
3. Auto-assisted shoulder flexion and elevation
4. Finger walking on the wall for shoulder abduction
5. Patient should be encouraged to do activities of daily livings
6. Rotation in sitting position with the arm by the side and elbow flexed to 90° during which ensures that there is no grinding sound produced.
7. As the pain subsides, weight and pulley exercises, theraband exercises and resisted exercises

Complications

1. Stiffness of the shoulder joint.
2. Axillary nerve injury
3. Associated fracture of greater tuberosity
4. Associated dislocation of shoulder.

FRACTURE OF SHAFT OF HUMERUS

Fracture of shaft of humerus usually occurs in adult at any age and rare in children. Fracture occurs due to fall on hand or on elbow.

Three types of fracture:

1. Spiral fracture occurs from rotational/twisting force.
2. Oblique or transverse fracture occurs from angular force.
3. Comminuted fracture occurs due to direct injury/blow.

The fracture heals readily because of good vascularity and clinically becomes stable within about 6 weeks. There is no tendency of over-riding, rather distraction by the weight of limb may cause delayed union. Spiral fracture may give rise to rotational malunion, interfering with functional actvities. Position of the greater tuberosity determines the neutral position of shoulder. With the shoulder in neutral position, orientation of cubital fossa and positions of the humeral epicondyles determine the rotational malunion. Medial rotation malunion of humeral shaft limit shoulder external rotation permanently. Angular deformity does not give rise to disability. Normally shaft of humerus is convex anteriorly, increase or decrease in normal anatomic angulation does not give rise to any problem. 20° of anterior angulation is accepted as muscle bulk masks the deformity.Frontal plane angulation may give rise to cubitus valgus or varus deformity.

Fracture involving the middle 1/3rd of the shaft may damage nutrient artery, which enters the bone at the junction of middle and lower 3rd medially affecting healing and results into delayed union or non-union. The radial nerve is at risk from fracture at the junction of middle and lower 3rd or operation of humerus. In most cases, the nerve is protected by a layer of triceps or brachialis muscle.

Management

The fractured ends whether oblique, transverse or spiral can be readily aligned by the weight of the limb with the patient sitting or standing. It requires supporting the wrist by collar and cuffing while the elbow is left free. In the early stage when there is considerable pain, a well padded plaster of paris U-slab passing down the outer side of the arm from the acromion and up the inner side to the region of the axilla bandanged with the trunk and supported by collar and cuff is effective in relieving discomfort. Once the initial discomfort subsides, the patient is encouraged to do active wrist and hand movements and static biceps, triceps contraction, which applies compression at the fracture site and stimulates osteogenesis. By keeping the hand within the collar and cuff, the patient leans forward, sideway and swings the arm for shoulder flexion-extension and abduction-adduction.

After removal of plaster, physiotherapy for relaxation of muscles around the joint, gradual mobilization and strengthening should be done.

Indication for primary operative management fracture:

1. Multiple fracture segments difficult to control by conservative means.
2. Multiple injuries associated with soft tissue injury, skin loss, etc.
3. Associated injury of the forearm, hand, etc. management of which becomes easy if humerus is fixed surgically.
4. Nonunion
5. Open fracture complicated by radial nerve injury following closed manipulative reduction under anesthesia.
6. Unstable fracture.

Intramedullary nail or compression plate screw fixation is done. For rigid fixation, heavy duty compression screw plate or closely fitting intramedullary nail must be used. Though IMN is easier, but for spiral or oblique fracture plate fixation is more effective. Intramedullary interlocking nail provides most rigid intramedulary immobilization. Nail introduced at the proximal end of humerus interferes with shoulder movements, usually introduced through distal humerus from olecranon.

Postoperatively in case of rigid fixation sling support is applied. Once initial acuteness subsides, active elbow, forearm and hand movements should be started. Graduated shoulder movements can be initiated earlier, shoulder rotation started after 7 days, so that full ROM is usually achieved by 2 weeks. In case, rigidity of fixation is in doubt, shoulder spica immobilization is applied for 4–6 weeks, during which active wrist and hand movements are encouraged.

After plaster removal, modality to relax muscles around shoulder joint is applied followed by graduated shoulder movements for strengthening and passive ROM exercises.

Radial nerve injury often recovers. Nerve injury following closed manipulative reduction and delayed gradual onset of nerve injury due to entrapment by callus requires surgical exploration for nerve repair or neurolysis.

SHOULDER DISLOCATION

Complete loss of contact between two articulating bones is known as dislocation whereas partial loss of contact is referred as subluxation. Incidence of anterior dislocation of shoulder is about 95% and posterior dislocation is about 5%.

Mechanism of Anterior Dislocation

External rotation and abduction injury gives rise to anterior dislocation, i.e. fall on outstretched hand or blow/fall on back of the shoulder, so that head of humerus is forced against the anterior capsule, which is therefore torn or avulsed from bone or glenoid labrum. The joint dislocates, the head may come to lie in front of the glenoid fossa of scapula, or if the force is stronger it is driven further forward to lie in the sub-coracoid or sub-clavicular position.

Tear of the capsule near the humeral attachment heals readily because of good vascularity, whereas tear of the capsule near the glenoid attachment is associated with injury to the glenoid labrum and the lesion is known as Bankart lesion. As the glenoid labrum is avascular, the healing is slow or incomplete resulting into re-dislocation.

Sometimes shoulder internal rotator, subscapularis, is avulsed from lesser tuberosity due to excessive stretching by external rotation injury. The greater tuberosity may be avulsed by the rotator cuff. During anterior dislocation, head may be impacted against the anterior margin the glenoid and gets fractured.

Complications

1. Injury to brachial plexus
2. Vascular injury

3. Rotator cuff injury.
4. Associated fracture greater tuberosity, lesser tuberosity, neck of humerus, head of humerus, glenoid rim (margin)
5. Recurrent dislocation

Clinical Features

The normal rounded contour of shoulder joint is lost. There is flattening of the shoulder and the acromion becomes prominent. Head lies in front of the glenoid fossa of scapula or below the coracoid process or below the clavicle. Movements in all directions are restricted.

Neurovascular examinations must be done before and after the reduction of dislocation. Lesion of the medial cord of brachial plexus is characterized by paralysis of small muscles of hand and loss of sensation on the medial aspect of hand and forearm. Lesion of posterior cord is characterized by paralysis of forearm extensors and wrist drop. Most commonly lateral cord and axillary nerves are injured. Injury to circumflex nerve is characterized by paralysis of deltoid. Muscle paralysis due to nerve injury must be differentiated from loss of function due to rotator cuff injury. Axillary vessels may be compressed or ruptured, which is characterized by loss of radial pulse. The hand may be cold and blue. Dislocation must be reduced promptly to relieve circulatory compromise.

Management

Closed manipulative reduction under anesthesia and immobilization with the shoulder in full medial rotation by axillary abduction pad and collar cuff sling is applied. The arm may be bandaged or strapped or simply incorporated under the vest, so that arm cannot move into external rotation and abduction for 3 weeks. By protecting the shoulder in medial rotation for 3 weeks, recurrence of dislocation is diminished.

During immobilization of active finger, wrist movements are encouraged from the beginning. Static contraction of deltoid, biceps, triceps and rotator cuff should be practiced.

Following reduction almost full JROM is present. Elevation of arm and combined shoulder abduction, lateral rotation should be avoided for 3 weeks to allow injured soft tissue to heal up. There is bruising and chance of synovitis to develop in elderly persons. Sling support is provided till the acute discomfort due to bruising and synovitis subsides. Apply ice 20 minutes 5 times/day for reabsorption of the exudates and relaxation of the spasm. Once initial discomfort subsides, active movements of elbow, forearm, wrist and hand should be encouraged. After 2–3 weeks, shoulder movements should be started. To start with shoulder rotatory movements, which move both the layers of the joint capsule to glide each other preventing adhesion formation. Codman's pendular exercises should be encouraged. Abduction beyond 90° and elevation through flexion should be avoided for 2–3 weeks. Gradual progressive strengthening of rotator cuff, biceps, triceps, coracobrachialis and deltoid should be done to prevent reccurence.

Late unreduced anterior dislocation is associated with adhesion and adoptive shortening of capsule, subscapularis muscle, axillary vein, artery and nerve. Attempted closed manipulative reduction may result into fracture of porotic bone, rupture of axillary vein or artery or traction injury of one of the cords of brachial plexus. In elderly persons, if there is no disability or complication due to late unreduced dislocation, it should be left like that. Young patients require operative reduction following which the arm is bandaged or strapped across the chest in medial rotation for 3 weeks.

Recurrent Anterior Dislocation of Shoulder

In young adults capsule is avulsed from the anterior margin of glenoid labrum. In elderly persons the capsule is ruptured about 2.5 cm proximal to the humeral attachment. Occasionally the capsule with the tendon of subscapularis is avulsed from the lesser tuberosity of humerus. If healing and repair of such injuries are not sound, recurrent anterior dislocation of shoulder may occur. The incidence is more in young men since the injured relatively hypovascular capsule does not heal properly. Associated fractures give rise to instability and recurrences. The incidence of recurrence reduces with post-reduction immobilization for 3 weeks.

Patient complains of recurrence from sudden lateral rotation and abduction of shoulder. Subsequent dislocations occur with increasing ease during combing, putting the sleeve of a coat, swimming, turning in bed, reaching over head, etc. activities.

Surgery

Putti-Platt operation involves repair and double breasting of anterior joint capsule and subscapularis. This procedure was first used by Sir Harry Platt of England and Vittorio Putti of Italy in 1920. Postoperatively the arm is immobilized in medial rotation for 3–4 weeks.

Postoperatively shoulder sling support is applied for 3–4 weeks, after which active ROM exercises are practiced. Isometric contractions of muscles and active movements are not allowed after operation, since muscles are cut and repaired. From 3–6 weeks, patients use the sling only during the night.

After 6 weeks, passive ROM exercises and gradual strengthening exercises should be encouraged. To start with eccentric followed by concentric exercises are given. More vigorous ROM exercises can be allowed after 8 weeks. Patient returns back to functional activities after 8–12 weeks.

BANKART

Anterior recurrent dislocation with healthy joint capsule and good vascularity to the glenoid labrum, the detached capsule and glenoid labrum are reattached to the front of the glenoid cavity. This procedure was first used by Bankart in 1923.

Postoperatively shoulder sling support is applied for 3-4 weeks, during which active fingers, wrist, forearm and elbow movements; and static contraction of rotator cuff, deltoid, biceps and, triceps are encouraged. After immobilization is removed, active ROM exercises, abduction up to 90 and external rotation to neutral position are practiced from 3–6 weeks. After

6 weeks, passive and active ROM exercises and gradual strengthening exercises should be encouraged.

Managing conservatively, the patients are advised to avoid combined abduction and external rotation, i.e. overhead activities.Internal rotators should be strengthened to relieve tension over anterior joint capsule and control external rotation.

Mechanism of Posterior Dislocation

Posterior dislocation of shoulder is uncommon. It occurs only in 5% cases due to vigorous internal rotation and adduction force usually occurs in epilepsy or electrical shock. Less commonly, it occurs by the direct blow from the front of the shoulder.

The capsule is torn or avulsed from the posterior margin of glenoid. There may be associated fracture, compression fracture of the head of humerus as it is impacted against the posterior margin of the glenoid. The head of humerus lies behind the scapula in a subspinous position. The normal rounded shoulder contour is lost and there is flattening. The arm is fixed in medially rotated position. All the movements are painful and restricted. Frequently missed on AP view X-ray shows almost normal.

Management

Closed manipulative reduction under anesthesia is achieved by traction in adduction and lateral rotation of arm. If the joint is stable after reduction as found by medially rotating the shoulder, a simple sling support for 2–3 weeks is provided. In case of persistent instability immobilization by shoulder spica with the arm in about 40° abduction and 30° lateral rotation is applied for 3 weeks.

Late unreduced posterior dislocation requires operative reduction through posterior approach. Postoperative immobilization depends on stability as determined at operation. If there is doubt, the arm is immobilized by shoulder spica with the arm in about 40° abduction and 30° lateral rotation for about 6 weeks.

Recurrent posterior dislocation of shoulder: Backward gliding of head of humerus during shoulder internal rotation displaces the head behind the glenoid. The capsule is detached with or without the glenoid labrum from the back of the joint. There may be associated fractures.

Operative procedure involves repair and double breasting of posterior joint capsule and infraspinatus. Postoperatively the arm is immobilized in plaster cast at about 40° medial rotation for 4 weeks.

ACROMIOCLAVICULAR JOINT INJURY

Stability of ACJ depends on the joint capsule reinforced by vertically oriented conoid ligament and horizontally oriented trapezoid ligament, parts of coracoclavicular ligament and the deltoid and trapezius muscles.

Mode of Injury

1. Fall on shoulder with arm adducted—common in football players.
2. Object falling on tip of shoulder.

Horizontal trapezoid ligament gives way first followed by vertical conoid ligament. Depending on severity of injury it is classified into three grades.

Grade I Sprain

Only a few fibers are disrupted. Anatomical and function integrity of the structure are maintained. Anatomical integrity is checked by stress test (P-A pressure, cephalocaudal pressure), whereas level of activities and disability determines the functional integrity. Localized tenderness present

Complaints of pain, well-localized at the shoulder tip, not referred down.

Pain is more during overhead activities or lifting or carrying weight. Amplitude of clavicular gliding is normal with little pain.

Management

Managed like soft issue lesion. No immobilization is required. Avoid precipitating movements and activities for 7–10 days.

Apply ice 20 minutes, 5 times per day. Progressive active range of motion exercises as pain allows applying optimal stress to injured structure should be encouraged. Progressive strengthening of deltoid and trapezius can be given after pain subsides reinforce stability of AC joint.

Grade II Sprain

Damage of horizontal fibers of coracoclavicular ligament gives rise to subluxation. Moderate A-P instability and mild vertical instability present. Impingement syndrome present and there will be impairment of overhead activities. Adduction, internal rotation of shoulder, i.e. placing the hand on opposite shoulder is painful. Applying downward distraction, step sign becomes positive.

Management

Arm is supported on a sling till pain subsides. Compression of acromioclavicular joint by applying Jones strapping. U-slab support compresses the joint from both up and down. The immobilization is given for 2–3 weeks.

Apply ice, as the acuteness subsides, active wrist and hand movements, and transverse friction massage, positional shoulder movements by leaning forward and sideways and static deltoid exercises are encouraged. Progressive strengthening of deltoid and trapezius and returns to activities after 3 weeks.

Grade III Sprain

All ligamentous structures are damaged giving rise to dislocation, characterized by typical step sign, i.e. acromion process is depressed downward by the weight of the limb and outer end of clavicle is elevated by the pull of trapezius and sternocleidomastoid. Normal contour of shoulder joint is lost.

Management

1. No treatment is given.

   To start with apply ice, rest is given to the part, isometric exercises as pain allows.

   Pain relieving modalities are applied followed by early movement and progressive strengthening.
2. Conservative management

   U-slab immobilization is given for 4–6 weeks. Ice, static exercises, active wrist and hand movements should be encouraged.

   After slab removal, graduated ROM and strengthening exercises of deltoid and trapezius should be given.
3. Operative management

   Acromioclavicular wiring or coracoclavicle screwing can be done.

Following screw fixation, early static exercises, after 7–8 days once stitch is removed, AROM exercises up to 90° and after 4–6 weeks progressive ROM and strengthening exercises can be started.

Following wiring, early static exercises and after 2–4 weeks active movements started. After 4–6 weeks progressive ROM and strengthening exercises can be started.

Late ACJ Injury

Reconstruction by using some fascia lata or conjoint tendon of coracobrachialis and short head of biceps can be done followed by immobilization for 6 weeks.

Complication:
- Impingement syndrome
- Unreduced dislocation
- Secondary osteoarthritis

STERNOCLAVICULAR JOINT INJURY

- Uncommon injury
- Caused by lateral compression of shoulder
- Anterior dislocation is most uncommon

The medial end of clavicle sometimes displaced upwards, rarely backwards. Swelling present due to synovitis. Retrosternal displacement presses over the trachea giving rise to dyspnea, greater vessels and traumatic shock, so it is a real emergency. In suspected cases airways and peripheral pulses must be assessed. It occurs due to head on collision in which the steering wheel pushes directly on the sternum and heart, direct blow to the front of clavicle or indirectly due to fall on shoulder. CT is ideal to comfirm the diagnosis.

Grade I sprain is characterized by mild to moderate pain during upper extremity movement. Localized tenderness, swelling present and there is no instability. Immobilized by sling for 3–4 days. Apply ice for 24 to 48 hours followed by heat and gradually return to activities.

Grade II sprain/subluxation is characterized by swelling, tenderness and pain during upper extremity movement. Immobilized by sling and apply ice for 24 to 48 hours followed by heat. Gradual strengthening of pectoralis minor and subclavius and gradually return to activities.

Grade III sprain/dislocation is characterized by pain increased by arm movement and compression on lateral aspect of shoulder. Patient feels discomfort when lying supine, supports the arm by the sound hand. The affected shoulder appears shortened and head tilted towards the side of dislocation. Medial clavicle becomes prominent.

The dislocation can be reduced by bracing the shoulder backwards, which can be maintained by figure of eight bandage with large axillary pad. It often redisplaces and requires surgery. In acute cases, torn ligaments are repaired. In late cases, repair must be reinforced with adjacent muscle and fascia or by stitching the meniscus of the joint across the front of the bone. Strips of fascia lata have been used to anchor the clavicle to the first or second rib or to the sternum. Unreduced SCJ dislocation may not cause any disability as the clavicle becomes stable in its displaced position without causing pain or limitation of motion.

BIBLIOGRAPHY

1. Craig EV: Fractures of the clavicle. In: Rockwood CA, Matsen FA (Editors): The shoulder, vol I, Philadelphia, Saunders 1990.
2. Dandy DJ: Essential orthopaedics and trauma, Edinburgh, Churchill Livingstone 1989.
3. Joshi J, Kotwal P. Essentials of orthopaedics and applied physiotherapy. Churchill Livingstone 1999.
4. Kisner C, Colby LA: Therapeutic exercise: foundations and techniques, edn 2, Philadelphia, FA Davis 1990.
5. Nettles JL, Linscheid R: Sternoclavicular dislocation J Trauma, 1968;8(2):158-64.
6. Peterson L, Renstrom P: Sports injuries: their prevention and treatment, London, Martin Dunitz 1986.
7. Rockwood CA, Matsen FA, (Editors): The shoulder, vol 1. Philadelphia, WB Saunders 1990.
8. Wale JO. Tidy's massage and remedial exercises in medical and surgical conditions. 11th edition. Wright: Bristol 1987.
9. Watson-Jones RR: Fractures and Joint Injuries. Vol 2, 4th edn. Baltimore, Williams and Wilkins, 1960.

Chapter 7

Myofascial Pain Syndrome

INTRODUCTION

Robert Froriep was the first to describe extremely tender, palpable hardening in muscles of patients with rheumatic disease in the year 1843. By the turn of the 20th century Adler associated the terms 'muscular rheumatism' with the concept of pain radiating from the tender spot in a muscle. In 1904, Gowers used the term 'Fibrositis' for the same symptom complex, but in a more specific sense and attributed the local tenderness and palpable hardness to inflammation of fibrous tissue. In 1919, Schade reported that the hardness of the previously tender ropiness persisted during deep anesthesia and even after death until it was obscured by diffuse rigor mortis. Later in 1921, he postulated a localized increase in viscosity of muscle colloid and proposed the term 'myogelosen', translated as "muscle gellings". In 1919, F Lange and G Eversbusch coined the term "Muskelharten" which means "Muscle hardenings", to describe tender points associated with regions of palpable hardness in skeletal muscle.

Hans Kraus, an early pioneer in this field, first reported the therapeutic use of ethyl chloride spray for relief of Muskelharten in 1937. There were no reports on the characteristic referred pain pattern till 1938, when Kellgren came out with his major milestone paper, which delineated referred pain pattern for major postural muscles when injected with saline. Shortly thereafter, these clinicians concurrently and independently published papers which had agreement in four cardinal features of myofascial trigger points. There were palpable hardness in the muscle, localized spot of tenderness, reproduction of the patient's complaint by digital pressure on the spot, and relief of pain by massage or injection of the tender spot. One of these studies, which was published in 1942, is regarded as the first of many studies published by Travell. Janet Travel published more than 40 papers on MTrPs between 1942 and 1990. Her two volumes of 'the trigger point manuals were published with Simons in 1983 and in 1992. In 1952, she and Rinzler reported the pain patterns of TrPs in 32 skeletal muscles as "the myofascial genesis of pain".

The word 'Fibrositis' was changed into fibromyalgia, which is defined as a condition of generalized pain marked by multiple tender points - by Yunus et al. In 1990, rheumatologist under the leadership of Wolfe officially established diagnostic criteria for fibromyalgia.

In the mid 1980's, Fischer introduced pressure algometry which is a quantitative method of measuring the sensitivity of MTrPs and of fibromyalgia tender points.

An important milestone of progress was reached by Hubbard and Berkoff in 1993 when they reported needle EMG activity characteristics of MTrPs. Recent studies had supported that a dysfunctional end plate region is the prime site of TrP pathophysiology.

PATHOPHYSIOLOGY

An important finding in the pathophysiology of myofascial pain is a pathologic increase in release of acetylcholine[7] by the nerve terminal of an abnormal motor endplate under resting condition. The acetylcholine is released to the synaptic cleft where it activates ACh receptors in the postjunctional membrane to produce increased numbers of miniature endplate potentials. These potentials are so numerous that they superimpose in order to produce endplate noise or spontaneous electrical activity (SEA) and a sustained postjunctional membrane depolarization. The excessive demand for production of ACh by the motor nerve terminal that would increase the energy demand. The increased activity at the postjunctional membrane and sustained depolarization further increases the energy demand.

The calcium channel that triggers release of calcium from the sarcoplasmic reticulum is voltage gated by depolarization of the T-tubule at the triad where the T-tubule communicates with the sarcoplasmic reticulum. The T-tubule is part of the same sarcolemmal membrane that forms the post-junctional membrane. This depolarization is one mechanism that might account for a tonic increase in the release of calcium from the sarcoplasmic reticulum to produce the local sarcomere contracture. This sustained release of calcium would increase the energy demand of the calcium pumps in the sarcoplasmic membrane. In summary the integrated hypothesis mentioned above is a positive feedback loop which starts with increased release of ACh at motor endplate due to mechanical trauma or chemical stimulation of the nerve terminal which induces a sustained sarcomere contraction. These results in localized ischemia, which in turn results in the release of substance that sensitizes nociceptors, produces pain, and induces release of neurovasoreactive chemicals. These chemicals lead to increase in ACh release sustaining the cycle.

Another hypothesis that was successful in explaining the pathophysiology of the TrP and its associated taut bands in the energy crisis hypothesis. Simons has explained this hypothesis in detail in a clinical commentary of a symposium entitled "Myofascial Triggers Points: Multidisciplinary Facets" presented at the 55th Annual Session of the American Congress of Rehabilitation Medicine on November, 1978. He later published an updated version in 1996. Mense has also contributed to our understanding of the neurophysiology of TrPs.

The energy crisis hypothesis postulates that an initial insult, such as mechanical rupture of either the sarcoplasmic reticulum or the sarcolemma, would release calcium that would maximally activate actin and myosin contractile activity. This together with the above discussed abnormal depolarization of the postjunctional membrane due to excessive ACh release. This results in a maximum indefinitely sustained contracture of the muscle fibers in the vicinity of the motor endpoint without motor unit action potential.

The sustained contractile activity of the sarcomere would markedly increase metabolic demands and squeeze shut the muscle off nutrition and oxygen. This combination of increased metabolic demand and impaired metabolic supply could produce a severe local energy crisis. The calcium pump that returns the calcium into sarcoplasmic reticulum also fails due to inadequate supply of ATP. Thus the contractile mechanism persists, assuring continued failure of the pump. When the ATP supply of the contractile mechanism is exhausted, a sustained contracture develops. In addition, the severe local hypoxia and tissue energy crisis could be expected to stimulate production of neurovasoreactive substances that sensitize local nociceptors.

Based on this hypothesis, the TrP region should (i) be higher in temperature than surrounding muscle tissue because of increase energy expenditure with impaired circulation to remove heat; (ii) be a region of significant hypoxia because of ischemia; (iii) have shortened sarcomeres.

One study by Travell in 1954 and another by Popelianskii et al in 1976, as reviewed by Simons and Mense recorded a focal increase in temperature in the region of the TrPs. One elegantly instrumented and validated study in German reported by the same authors examined affected muscle for focal hypoxia and encountered remarkably positive results. The examiners used a sensor and found that the tissue oxygen tension fell abruptly to nearly zero, indicating profound hypoxia in the central region of the induration. Simons and Stolov in their study on canine muscles by doing biopsy of those containing tender spot and taut bands found multiple contraction knots with increased diameter.

A recent study reported by Simons also found similar morphological changes in the palpable nodules. The examiner biopsied, from fresh cadavers, palpable nodules present in the gluteus medius muscle. Cross-sections showed the previously described, large rounded muscle fibers and a statistically significant increase in the average diameter of muscle fibers in the palpable nodules.

The combined tension produced by multiple contraction knots may account for the increased palpable tension of the taut band. The unrelieved sustained tension of muscle fibers in the taut band produces an enthesopathy at their myotendinous junction that can be identified as an attachment MTrPs.

The localized muscle ischemia stimulates the release of neurovasoreactive substances such as prostaglandin, bradykinin, capsaicin, serotonin and histamine that sensitize afferent nerve fibers in muscle. These sensitized fibers in turn account for local MTrP tenderness.

The basis for the electrodiagnostic approach to the study of MTrPs was anticipated by Weeks and Travell in 1957. They reported that TrPs in the resting trapezius muscle exhibited a series of high frequency spike shaped discharge while the adjacent sites in the muscle were electrically silent. This study was followed by Hubbard and Berkoff who demonstrated the presence of "spontaneous EMG activity" at minute sites in an MTrP region of the upper trapezius muscle. This continuous low amplitude activity was defined as SEA. The minute needle sites from which spikes only, SEA only, or both may appear is defined as active locus.

The potentials found at the active loci of TrPs corresponded completely to the potential that are recognized by electromyographers as normal motor end plate potential. An early literature reviewed by Hong and Liley reported an abnormal pattern of endplate potentials similar to SEA when the endplate was mechanically disturbed. Additionally, chemical stimulation of normal endplates may produce an endplate noise pattern at as much as 1000 times the normal rate of spontaneous discharge. Ito et al demonstrated that this abnormal pattern of endplate potential was attributed to excessive release of ACh. It is therefore possible that mechanical, chemical or other noxious stimuli or injury may mediate the abnormal release of ACh. At this point it became necessary for us to think that the SEA and spikes characteristics of active loci in symptom-producing TrPs represented normal endplate activity.

CENTRAL MECHANISMS

The referred pain from the TrP arises from central convergence and facilitation. It is known from experimental data that, under pathologic conditions, convergent connections from deep afferent nociceptors to dorsal horn neurons are facilitated and amplified in the spinal cord. Referral to adjacent myotomes occurs due to spreading of central sensitization to adjacent spinal segments. This pattern results in both referred pain and in expansion of the region of pain beyond the initial nociceptive region.

At the level of the central nervous system, spinal neuroplastic changes occur in the second-order neuron pool of the dorsal horn due to persistent pain. These changes produce a long lasting increase in the excitability of the nociceptor pathways which include increased excitability of the neurons and expansion of the receptive pool of neurons. Neurotransmitters involved in the process of central sensitization include substance-P, N-methyl-D-aspartate, glutamate and nitric oxide. In addition, there may be impairment in supraspinal inhibitory descending pain control pathways.

AUTONOMIC NERVOUS SYSTEM

Several studies have supported the notion of sympathetic nervous system innervation to muscle, in particular, the intrafusal fibers of the muscle spindle. This is in contrast with traditional views that skeletal muscle is innervated only by the voluntary nervous system. This led Passatore and his colleagues to speculate that some aspects of muscle tension are actually mediated by intrafusal contraction of the muscle spindle. The clinical observation of autonomic phenomenon associated with active MTrPs has been well documented. The prevalence of MTrPs in reflex sympathetic dystrophy and its influence on the treatment outcomes of RSD is previously established. The observations that psychological stress intensifies both TrP pain and the electrical activity at the active loci of TrPs fit clinical experience and experimental evidence. Schwatrz et al compared multiphasic personality profiles of successfully treated MPS patients with unsuccessfully treated counterparts and found that the later group had a higher degree of emotional distress.

Under pathologic conditions, the neurovasoreactive substances such as bradykinin, substance P, serotonin and histamine also stimulates activity of the local ANS fibers to release more ACh, completing the positive feedback loop of integrated hypothesis. McNulty et al stated that end plate spike rate increasing by psychological stress. Spike activity was inhibited in human and rabbit by administering a-sympathetic blockers. Thus there seems to be a relationship between autonomic activation and increased motor endpoint activity. The relationship of emotional and psychological factors to MTrP sensitivity has also been commented.

There are authors who even question the existence of myofascial pain. Johnson suggests that measuring pain with quantitative methods is only half of the story. He also gives less importance to the nociceptive impulse from the soft tissue. Whereas, he believes that there are innumerable possibilities at the CNS level which will determine the final outcome. These include memory of pain, state of activation of CNS, culture, significance of pain, personal characteristics and economic prospects.

TRIGGER POINT IN MYOFASCIAL PAIN SYNDROME (MPS)

Myofascial pain syndrome (MPS) as a term has acquired both a general and a specific meaning, which needs to be distinguished. The general meaning includes a regional muscle pain syndrome of any soft tissue origin that is associated with muscle tenderness. Myofascial trigger points (MTrPs) can be defined as a hyperirritable locus within a taut band of skeletal muscle that is painful to palpation, reproduce the patients symptoms, and cause referred pain.

The prevalence of MPS has been increasing dramatically in recent years. Skootsky et al examined a series of 172 patients presenting to a university primary care general internal medicine practice and found that out of 54 patients who recently included pain, 30% satisfied criteria for a clinical diagnosis of myofascial pain. This percentage is probable underestimating the incidence because it is probably based on the narrower definition of myofascial pain limited to the Trigger Points that induce symptoms in the referred pain zone (RPZ). If tender spots, which cause local pain in the area of maximal tenderness, are also considered, then myofascial pain is certainly the most frequent immediate cause or component of musculoskeletal pain. The mean intensity of pain of the patients diagnosed as having myofascial pain as assessed by the visual analogue scale, was comparable to or possibly greater than the intensity of other pain complaints that brought study patients to see their physician. TrPs were the primary source of pain in 85% of 283 patients consecutively admitted to a comprehensive pain centre. Fifty five percentage of 164 patients referred to a dental clinic for chronic head and neck pain were found to have active MTrPs as the cause of their pain. Fischer reviewed a prevalence study in Myofascial pain in non-patient control groups and indicated that 54% females and 45% males demonstrated focal tenderness indicative of latent TrPs in the shoulder girdle muscles in a young population. Recent study shows that myofascial pain is present in all patients with cumulative trauma disorders and the treatment of TrPs or tender spots improved the rate of success substantially in this category of patients. Similarly, 82% of patients suffering from reflex sympathetic dystrophy demonstrated myofascial pain and treatment of the tender spots and TrPs component improved the outcome of this difficult condition.

These epidemiological studies suggest that MTrP pain is an important source of morbidity in the community. The associated autonomic dysfunctions including abnormal sweating, lacrimation, dermal flushing and temperature changes makes the diagnosis and management issues more complicated. Cervical myofascial pain may be associated with neurologic symptoms including imbalance dizziness and tinnitus. Other associated neurologic symptoms include paresthesia, numbness, blurred vision, twitches and trembling. Clinically, persons with cervical MPS have a very high recurrence rate. Upper trapezius is the muscle that most frequently contains trigger points and almost always contributes to head and neck pain complaints. Upper trapezius trigger points may also be one of the most painful sites as there is a tendency for points in the nape region to have the lowest pressure pain threshold. The high predilection for tender points in the upper middle area of the trapezius may be due to the fact that it contains fewer mitochondria per volume of muscle fibers than other muscle. The mid-trapezius area also marks the critical angle of neck lateral bending and postural fixation for movements of the arm, which result in increased tension.

Simons et al have hypothesized that the pathophysiology of the MFPS and formation of TrPs results from an injured or overstressed muscle fibers, leading to tightness and loss of oxygen and nutrient supply with increased metabolic demand on local tissue - Energy crisis hypothesis. The excessive release of intracellular calcium in certain muscles and a pathologic increase in release of acetylcholine (Ach) by the nerve terminal of an abnormal motor endplate is supported by electrodiagnostic evidence and this abnormality is considered to be the primary dysfunction in the "integrated hypothesis" proposed by Simons and Mense. Their hypothesis has been supported by studies that showed a low oxygen tension in the MTrPs region and a significant decrease in high energy phosphates coupled with an increase in low energy phosphates and creatine in a tender muscle site. Some authors are of the opinion that TrP may result from or be irritated by trauma, overuse, mechanical load, postural faults or psychological stress.

MTrP mechanism is closely related to the spinal cord integration. When the input from the nociceptors in an original receptive field persists, central sensitization in the spinal cord may develop and the receptive field corresponding to the original dorsal horn neuron may be expanded. Through this mechanism new MTrPs or satellite MTrPs may develop in the referred pain zone. Researchers have successfully treated satellite TrPs by injection therapy to the primary trigger point. For a long-standing untreated active MTrP, the irritation from the peripheral nociceptors may be persistant and the expansion of receptive field may increase progressively. Finally spontaneous pain may spread to many distant regions in addition to the original reference zone through the mechanism of central sensitization in the spinal cord. A latent trigger point is clinically silent with respect to pain, but may cause decreased extensibility and weakness of that muscle. The patient may not be aware of the latent trigger point until the clinician compresses it and the patient experiences local pain or referred pain.

Travell and Simons formulated a list of generalized clinical characteristics of trigger points:

1. Trigger point is a hyperirritable focus present within the taut band of the skeletal muscle, compression of which reproduces local pain and referred pain.
2. Autonomic disturbances such as abnormal sweating, lacrimation, salivation, pilomotor activity, dermal flushing and temperature changes, etc. may be seen in the referred region.
3. Stretching of the involved muscle reproduces the symptoms and there is loss of extensibility.
4. Resisted isometric contraction of involved muscle reproduces the symptoms and there is weakness.

TRIGGER POINT IN FIBROMYALGIA (FM)

The most common and most disabling feature that patients report is a diffuse and burning pain over wide areas of body affecting primarily the torso but head, neck and extremities as well. This is accompanied by a severe stiffness when the patient remains in one position for a prolonged period of time, but is most severe in the morning upon arising. Fatigue is another symptom. Other common symptoms are headache, jaw and face pain, short-term memory loss, difficulty in swallowing, irritable bowel syndrome, burning pain in extremities and arthralgias of small joints of hands and feet. Sometimes other systems such as cardiac, dermatologic, genitourinary, gynecologic and dental are involved. Depression is a common problem and often interpreted as the cause rather than the effect. The history and appropriate laboratory investigations should be done to rule out collagen vascular disease and thyroid disease.

The characteristic features of fibromyalgia as defined by the American Rheumatism Association are 18 tender points bilaterally symmetrically distributed in the body (suboccipital muscle insertion, anterior aspects of intertransverse spaces at C5-7, trapezius at the midpoint of upper border, supraspinatus, 2nd costochondral junctions, lateral epicondyles of humerus, gluteus upper and outer quadrants, greater trochanter, anteromedial aspect of knee and the presence of abnormalities in 11 of these is necessary to establish the diagnosis (Fig. 7.1). Widespread diffuse pain lasting at least 3 months.

Myofascial Pain Syndrome (MPS) and Fibromyalgia (FM)

Myofascial Pain Syndrome (MPS) and Fibromyalgia (FM) were seen as separate clinical entity both in the aspects of pathophysiology and clinical manifestation in the early 90's. The distance between these two conditions is becoming nearer, both in the pathogenesis and its occurrence. Hong cited studies by Bennet, which stated that the pathogenesis of tender points in fibromyalgia syndrome and trigger points in MFPS, are

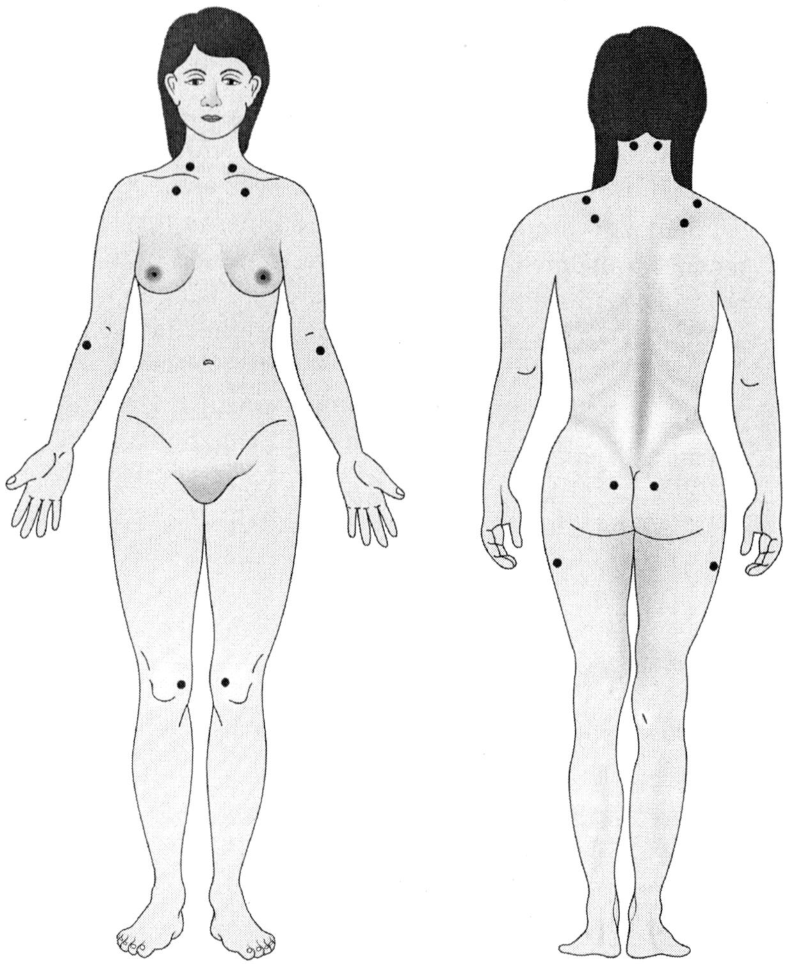

Fig. 7.1: Tender points in fibromyalgia as defined by American Rheumatism Association

exactly the same. Both the investigators emphasized that, in their clinical practice, almost every patient with fibromyalgia syndrome has diffuse trigger points. They stated that a tender point in the muscle is the same as a trigger point. The only difference in the pain mechanism is that the pain threshold is severely and diffusely reduced in many tissues in FM. This apparently results from biochemical disorders in the central nervous system. The common features of MPS and FM are fatigue, poor sleep, depression, anxiety, negative laboratory findings, neurologic evaluation and joint examination, pain increased on stress, tension and strenuous exercise or activities, pain decreased by local heat application and mild exercise.

Patient's own complaints are reproduced by pressure over the trigger points in myofascial pain syndrome (MPS). Caused by acute muscle strain or chronic overuse of specific group of muscles. Male to female ratio is equal. Local tender point present, pressure pain threshold of which is decreased and compression of which reproduced original symptoms. In fibromyalgia (FM) pain is diffuse, not reproduced by pressure over the trigger point. Insidious onset of generalized pain and often fatigue. It occus mostly in females. Tenderness over 11 points out of 18 is diagnostic of fibromyalgia.

Trigger Points and Tender Points

Pressure threshold, which is the minimum pressure that induces pain is considered abnormal if it is lower by 2 kg/cm relative to the normosensitive control point which is usually measured over the opposite side. All tender points are not trigger points. Trigger point is that tender point which reproduces patient's symptoms on digital pressure over it. Infiltration by local anesthesia abolishes the pain.

SKELETAL CHANGES

Joint dysfunction often coexists with the myofacial pain syndrome. Considerable controversies exist as to whether the primary problem resides in the muscles or the joint. Joint dysfunction and soft tissue problems may be primary or secondary. If primary, an attempt should be made to eradicate them. If secondary, they should be treated along with the primary problem. Although one can readily understand that problem is a neurologic one with false signals being sent to the muscles which then goes into spasm and causes loss of motion of the joint (David A John). Korr and associates demonstrate that decreased pain threshold, increased sympathetic activity and facilitation of motor pathways, associate with articular dysfunction. They reported a marked increase in paraspinal muscle activity associated with dysfunctional articular segment (Mense and Simons).

Joints are meant to move through a full painless range of motion. Whether the pathology is within or without the joint, the resultant decrease in range of motion produces pain. A muscle is meant to contract fully and relax fully. Failure to do so results in the accumulation of catabolites and results in pain. Soft tissues are meant to glide painlessly—one over the other. Failure to do so results in pain. The vascular and lymphatic systems are meant to empty fully. Failure to do so results in stasis, edema and interference with proper functioning of the musculoskeletal system. It can then be seen that the final common path is loss of range of motion and resultant pain. When faced with such problems, all must be corrected before pain is relieved. When that has been accomplished, the final step is the restoration of strength by a progressive exercise program.

MANAGEMENT

Despite the improved understanding of the pathophysiological mechanism of MPS due to histopathologic and electrodiagnostic studies, efficacy of treatment modalities to alleviate the pain and discomfort is not well established. The major goal of MTrP therapy is to relieve pain and tightness of the involved muscles. Traditional treatment techniques include ischemic compression, acupressure, deep pressure soft tissue massage, post-isometric relaxation and myofascial release in the form of manual therapy. Cryotherapy/Vapocoolant spray is used to augment the passive stretch and was recommended by Travell and Simons. This treatment method is slowly getting discarded from the field of myofascial therapy because of the suspected effects of fluorimethane—the vapocoolant used as the spray—

on the ozone layer. Electrotherapy treatment includes therapeutic ultrasound, TENS and other electrical stimulation.

TENS works as per pain gate theory for pain modulation. Faradism under tension can be used to stretch the fibrosed muscles. IFT relieves the pain, improves circulation and increases the extensibility of the involved muscle. Ultrasound (US) is a common treatment modality that has traditionally been used by the physiotherapist for the treatment of MTrPs because of its deep heating effects with added benefits of its non-thermal properties.

Aerobics exercises stimulate the body's own pain inhibiting mechanism by increasing endorphin and enkephalin. The stretching techniques used in the conventional treatment was described by Lewit K. well-known as post-isometric relaxation and is a form of muscle energy technique. Travell and Simons have recommended this technique as an effective adjunct to myofascial therapy. This technique includes taking the muscle to the point of taking a slack, doing a submaximal isometric contraction and relaxing it and augmenting the relaxation using coordinated breathing techniques.

Ischemic compression (IC) as described by Travell and Simons is the application of sustained pressure to the trigger point. The pressure is progressed as the pain of the trigger point abates. Recent studies have shown that IC with the pressure same as the pain threshold with duration of 90 sec. was effective in treating MTrPs. Hanten et al found that IC and sustained stretching was effective in reducing the TrPs sensitivity and pain intensity in patients having MPS. Similar variants of IC like acupressure and deep pressure soft tissue massage was also found to be effective for the treatment of TrPs. The mechanisms which may explain the efficacy of this manual therapy includes 'neurological overload', the release of endogenous morphine like products (endorphins, enkephalins) as well as 'flushing' of tissues with fresh oxygenated blood following the compression.

ULTRASOUND

Ultrasound is found to heat tissues with high collagen content, such as Tendon, ligament, or fascia and, for the past 50 years or more has been widely used in the clinical setting for this purpose. The thermal and non-thermal properties of US have been traditionally considered separately. Continuous US has the most effect on tissue temperature; however, non thermal effects can also occur with the use of continuous US. The thermal effects include pain reduction, increased perfusion decreased muscle spasm, increase in collagen extensibility and alternation of nerve conduction velocity. These therapeutic effects are same as those of other heating modalities, except that the depth of heating and structures heated varies. Typically, 1 MHz US in the continuous mode is used for heating tissue 2.5 – 5 cm deep, whereas 3 MHz is used to heat tissues less than 2.5-cm deep. Tissues with high absorption coefficients are generally those with high collagen content and thus are suited to heat tendon, ligament, joint capsule and fascia.

For the majority of the thermal effects of US to occur, the temperature should increase to a therapeutic range of 40°C to 45°C. Other studies, reported that a 1°C rise of temperature from the baseline increases metabolism and healing, 2°C to 3°C decreases pain and muscle spasm and 4°C or greater increases the extensibility of collagen and decrease joint stiffness. Based on calculation by Draper 1 MHz US at 2.5 W/cm^2 for 3 minutes (2ERA) would increase tissue temperature only 1.2°C. The increase in temperature depends on duration and intensity of insonation. Out of the 10 studies accepted by Robertson for the review, used pulsed mode for insonation. Thus they have failed to heat the tissues by not taking into consideration the size of the treatment area, duration of insonation, frequency of the treatment head and percentage of sonation. The two studies that showed that active US is superior than placebo, had the longest treatment time of 15 minutes. Therefore any study which addresses the clinical efficacy of US should strictly adhere to all these parameters which is scientific.

Evidence in support of the US for the treatment of MTrPs is mixed. Five studies are confronted out of which 3 supported 2 contrary to and 1 neutral about the use of US for the treatment of myofascial pain.

Lee Lin and Hong did a study on the immediate effects of US and electrical stimulation compared to electrical stimulation only for the treatment of MTrPs. They found that the range of stretch of upper trapezius muscle was significantly increased immediately after the application of US and electrical stimulation compared to the group, which received electrical stimulation alone. Esposito et al and Talaat et al also supports the use of US for the treatment of MPS. Esposito evaluated the effects of US on 28 patients and found that it was effective in alleviating discomfort of MPS that does not respond to occlusal splint therapy used in dentistry. Talaat studied a population of 120 patients who have MPS who were randomly assigned into three equal groups treated by muscle relaxant drugs, short wave diathermy, and US therapy respectively. This was a long-term study with regular follow up for 6–12 months. Results revealed marked relief of symptoms by the use of physiotherapy and the best results were obtained by the use of ultrasonic therapy.

Gam et al investigated the effect of ultrasound, massage and exercise on MTrPs. This was a long-term study and fifty eight patients who had TrPs in the neck and shoulder were divided into three groups. The first group was treated with massage, exercise and US; the second with same US, massage and exercise and the third was a control group. Duration of the study was 6 weeks and a long-term carry over was checked by using a questionnaire sent to the patients after 6 months of the last treatment session. The authors did not find any difference between the experimental groups and the control group and thus concluded that US gives no pain reduction, but apparently massage and exercise reduces the number and intensity of MTrP. The outcome measures in this study were

VAS, a tender point score with three points, daily analgesic use and a follow up questionnaire for long-term effects. The reliability of the tender point score and the analgesic usage as a treatment outcome measure is questionable. No algometer was used to measure the individual trigger point sensitivity.

The US frequency they used was 1MHz, Pulse mode 2:8, 3 W/cm^2 for 3 minutes. Technical details regarding the ERA are not mentioned even though it is mentioned that the radiation area was 0.8 cm^2. Using 1MHz was an ideal decision because of the increased depth of penetration, but using pulsed mode with a mark space ratio of 2:8 delivering only 20% of the US energy lacks empirical support. The thermal effects of pain reduction, increased perfusion decreased spasm increase in the extensibility of the fascia, which has more of collagen and alternation in nerve conduction velocity may have an effect on the painful, hypoxic, tense MTrP. As the output of the US was pulsed no thermal effect would have occurred. Provided the fact that thermal dose can also cause non-thermal effects there was no need of a pulsed output. The tissue temperature should increase to more than 40°C for therapeutic benefits and it depends upon the duration of insonation also. Draper's study has proved that insonation using continuous mode, 1 MHz treatment head at an intensity of 2.5 W/cm^2 for 3 minutes (2ERA) would increase tissue temperature only 1.2°C. So this study despite using 3W/cm^2 would not have reached the therapeutic range because of pulsed mode and shorter treatment time. Thus Gam failed to use contemporary US methodologies rooted in experimental literature.

Esenyel et al in his recent study on myofascial pain investigated the effectiveness of US treatment and trigger point injection in combination with neck stretching exercises on myofascial TrPs of the upper trapezius muscle. One hundred and two patients were randomly assigned into one of three groups: group 1 received US therapy to the TrPs in conjunction with neck stretching exercises; group 2 received TrP injection and neck stretching exercises; and group 3, the control group, performed neck stretching exercises only. Outcome measures were VAS for subjective pain intensity, algometer for pressure pain threshold and a goniometer for ROM of the upper trapezius muscle. This too was a long-term study with follow up for 3 months. In the conclusion, the authors reported that when combined with neck stretching exercises, US treatment and TrP injections were found to be equally effective.

The authors should be appreciated for their effort to assess the psychological status of the patients using the Beck depression inventory and the Taylor manifest anxiety scale. As the relationship of emotional and psychological factors is well established and sympathetic contribution is well proved in the case of MTrPs, this was a very appropriate and timely step taken by the authors. But the US parameters used had flaws in it. The intensity of US was 1.5 W/cm^2 for 6 minutes duration. This could be an acceptable dosage if the treatment was twice the size of ERA. Instead the authors reported that they sonated the trigger point as well as the pain referral zone for a total time of 6 minutes. Pain referral zone of the upper trapezius is found to be extending to the side of the head and posterolateral part of the neck as well as the angle of the jaw. This duration of US application is in contrary with Draper's research findings and Robbins' recommendation regarding sonation of a TrP.

From all the studies reviewed, Hong's study was one among those which compared a variant of ischemic compression with US therapy. Hong compared four modalities i.e; stretch and spray, moist heat, US and deep pressure soft tissue massage and found that all four modalities were effective in the treatment of MPS and deep pressure massage therapy was the most effective modality. Robbins had critically appraised Hong's study and stated that the results are highly inconsistent with his clinical experience. He states that the unexpected results may be due to rapid movement of the US head and large area covered during a small duration of 5 minutes. Robbin's based his arguments on Dr Lowe's teaching of ultrasound treatment of the TrPs. Hong states that US was applied to the upper trapezius area of approximately 40–50 cm^2 with the TrP at the central portion with an intensity of 1.2– 1.5 W/cm^2 for a duration of 5 minutes. He moved the ultrasound head 3–5 cm/sec and made sure that the patients always felt warm during therapy.

The intensity of 1.2–1.5 W/cm^2 would have been an effective dosage if the duration was more. There are studies which proved in vivo that when 1 MHz US was given with gel as a coupling medium with 1.5 W/cm^2 intensity in a continuous mode took 8 minutes to heat the tissues to a therapeutic level of 40°C. This temperature rise was when 2 ERA was insonated with the head moving 4cm/sec. Thus it is unlikely that the area covered by Hong (40–50 cm^2) reaches the therapeutic range of temperature. It is also shown that the movement of the transducer head should be 2–3 cm/sec for optimal results.

All the other methodology used by Hong for the application of US is acceptable as per the recent research findings. The intensity of more than 1 W/cm^2 delivered with a continuous mode has been proved to increase temperature and blood flow. The speed of movement of the US head was also not far from the recommended speed of 2–3 cm. Hong has attempted to get a feedback of warmth during the US treatment. This is supported by authors who suggest that the patient should feel a heating sensation with effective thermal US treatment.

POST-ISOMETRIC RELAXATION (PIR)

PIR refers to the effect of the subsequent reduction in tone experienced by a muscle, or group of muscle, after brief periods during which an isometric contraction has been performed. Karel Lewit has reported on the usefulness aspects of Muscle Energy Technique (MET) in the treatment of TrPs. This is seen by many to be an excellent method of treating this myofascial status, and of achieving the restoration of a situation where the muscle in which the TrP lies is once more capable of achieving its full resting length, with no evidence of shortening.

Travell and Simons mistakenly credited Lewit with developing MET, but it is acknowledged by Lewit that Mitchell,

Sr. pioneered this mobilization technique. The techniques involve taking the muscle to a length just short of pain, the patient contracting the muscle for 5–10 sec. with an inhalation, the therapist preventing the shortening of the muscle followed by the patient relaxing the muscle with an exhalation.

Lewit and Simons have investigated the effectiveness of PIR in a large population having MTrPs. They treated 351 muscles of 244 patients and reported that the method produced immediate pain relief in 94%, lasting pain relief in 63%, as well as lasting pain relief of point tenderness in 23% of the sites treated. They recommended this technique in addition to, or in place of local anesthetic injection or dry needling. The outcome measure of this study seems to be only subjective and there was no control group in this study.

Jaeger and Reeves quantified the changes in MTrP sensitivity with a pressure algometer after passive stretch and spray of the involved muscle. They found that TrP sensitivity decreased in response to passive stretch. They did not compare their findings with a control group and the sample size was small consisting of 20 patients. This study was one among the pioneer studies, which used algometer as the outcome measure.

The effects of PIR may be due to the following facts:

- During resistance using minimal force only a few muscle fibers are active, the other being inhibited.
- During relaxation (in which the shortened musculature is taken gently to its new limit without stretching) the stretch reflex is avoided - a reflex which may be brought about even by passive and non-painful stretch.

ISCHEMIC COMPRESSION

Direct inhibitory pressure has a long history of use in many forms of bodywork including osteopathy in order to achieve a release of hypertonically tense tissue, spasm and cramp. Dr Raymond Nimmo, a chiropractor and Bonnie Pruden a massage therapist, described ischemic compression being the most effective way to treat a TrP.

The term 'ischemic compression' is replaced by the new term "trigger point pressure release (TPPR)" for two reasons. No experimental evidence substantiates ischemia as the primary mechanism for the effectiveness of this technique, and therapists have been prone to apply unnecessarily excessive force, which can be counter productive and painful to the patients. The technique now recommended conform to the concept of barrier release. Gentle gradually increasing pressure is applied until the barrier is encountered and it is maintained till the barrier releases. Travell and Simons recommend duration up to 1-minute with as much as 20 or 30 lb of pressure. The technique promoted by some chiropractors employs pressure for only 7–10 second.

One recent study by Hou et al compared 30 sec, 60 sec and 90 sec duration of TPPR with two pressure loading; pain threshold and averaged value of pain threshold and pain tolerance. He found that the lower pressure at pain threshold level for duration of 90 sec was effective in obtaining pain relief. The pressure that is applied to the MTrP of taut band should be within a tolerable pain level for individual patients to avoid causing excessive pain and autonomic responses with involuntary muscle tensing. The treatment may not be effective if insufficient pressure is applied. Therefore, an appropriate pressure prescription is important to ensure the clinical efficacy of TPPR therapy. A quantified delivery of pressure for a specific duration to the TrP also ensures replicability of the same method in clinical practice or controlled trials. Even though algometers were extensively used for the outcome measure of myofascial therapy, it has been rarely used as a measure to quantify the delivered pressure during IC to a MTrP.

Hou's study was comparing the immediate effects of physiotherapy on cervical myofasical pain and TrP sensitivity and compared six combinations of seven therapeutic modalities i.e; hot pack, active ROM, IC, TENS, stretch and spray, IFT and myofascial release. They found that immediate relief can be obtained in all combinations and the most effective was the combination of hot packs plus active ROM, IC, and TENS. It was not clear whether the immediate effect was attributed to IC or TENS. The long-term effects of these modalities were not considered in this study. There was a need to investigate the long-term effectiveness of TPPR after a quantified delivery of pressure which is equal to the PPT for a duration which was found most effective by Hou et al.

Hanten et al conducted a study on forty adults with MPS and compared the effect of a home program of IC followed by sustained stretching with a control treatment of active ROM. The IC group demonstrated the effectiveness of IC in reducing TrP sensitivity as measured by algometer and pain intensity scored with a VAS. The idea of giving a type of manual therapy like IC as a home program is defended by the statement, "We believe that the patient should be involved in his or her treatment, acting as the primary pain manager". Another advantage of home program is that it reduces physiotherapy visits. The study was not designed to distinguish the relative contribution of IC from those of stretching exercises. The reliability of MTrP examination has been strongly criticized by other authors. Wolfe et al conducted a reliability study of TrP examination on four experts on MPS and found problems with reliability for taut bands, muscle twitch and active TrPs. Nice et al did a study to determine the inter tester reliability of assessment of the presence of TrPs by physiotherapist and found that reliability was less. Marginal kappa value of 10.49 was reached only when the examiners are trained for the examination. Given the fact that TrP identification has less reliability, the patient finding the taut band and the trigger point and applying IC consistently for 5 days using a theracane in a successful manner is questionable. Hypersensitive patients also may tend not to press at a site where they have more pain.

Garvey et al compared the effect of injection of a local anesthetic, injection of a local anesthetic plus steroid, acupuncture and acupressure with vapocoolant spray on MTrPs. The authors found that the acupressure plus vapocoolant sprays, their control procedure was the most effective at relieving pain.

Some authors identify the acupressure as ischemic comparison.

Hong et al evaluated the immediate effects of four commonly used modalities used by physiotherapist who treat MTrPs. The modalities they tested included stretch and spray, moist heat, ultrasound, and deep pressure soft tissue massage. The investigators wrote that also four modalities were effective in the treatment of MPS and deep pressure soft tissue massage was the most effective modality.

The efficacy of applied compression may be attributed to:

- Decreasing of hypertonicity, apparently by releasing the contracted sarcomeres in the TrP nodule.
- A mechanical stress on the colloidal matrix, which may alter its state from that of a gel to sol.
- The over-riding of neural reflex mechanism, thereby reducing spasm through gating mechanism.
- Blanching to tissues, which is followed by flushing of blood that brings oxygen and nutrients.
- Release of endorphins and enkephalins.
- Neurologic inhibition that is achieved by means of the sustained barrage of efferent information resulting from the constant pressure.
- Alternation of energy flow along hypothesized meridians according to the acupuncture and acupressure concepts.

Subscapularis (Fig. 7.2)

In supine lying position arm abducted to 90° and elbow flexed to 90°, external rotation of shoulder stretches the subscapularis.

Teres Minor (Fig. 7.3)

In side lying position elevation of arm behind the head with depression of scapula stretches the teres minor muscle.

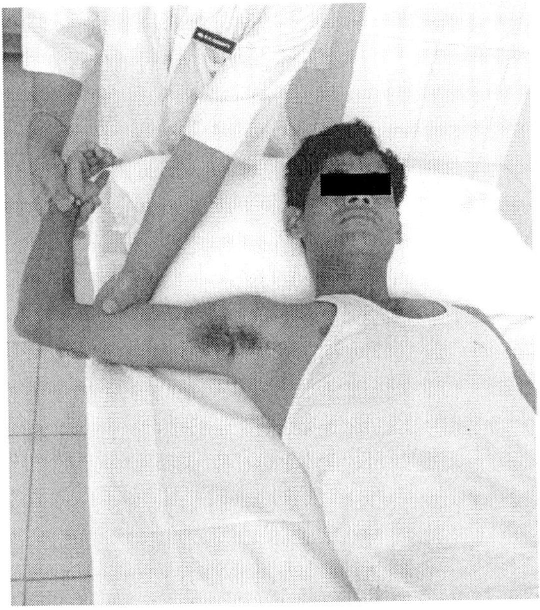

Fig. 7.2: Stretching of subscapularis

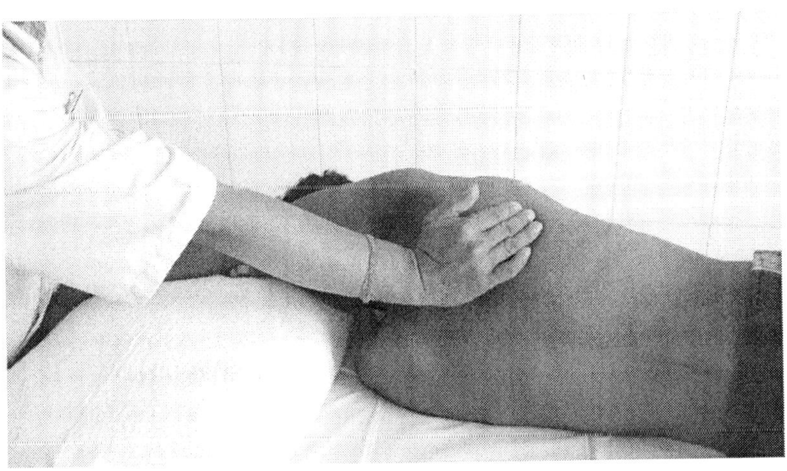

Fig. 7.3: Stretching of teres minor

Teres Major (Fig. 7.4)

In supine lying position with the arm elevated elbow flexed and hand under the head, press the elbow towards the couch to stretch the teres major.

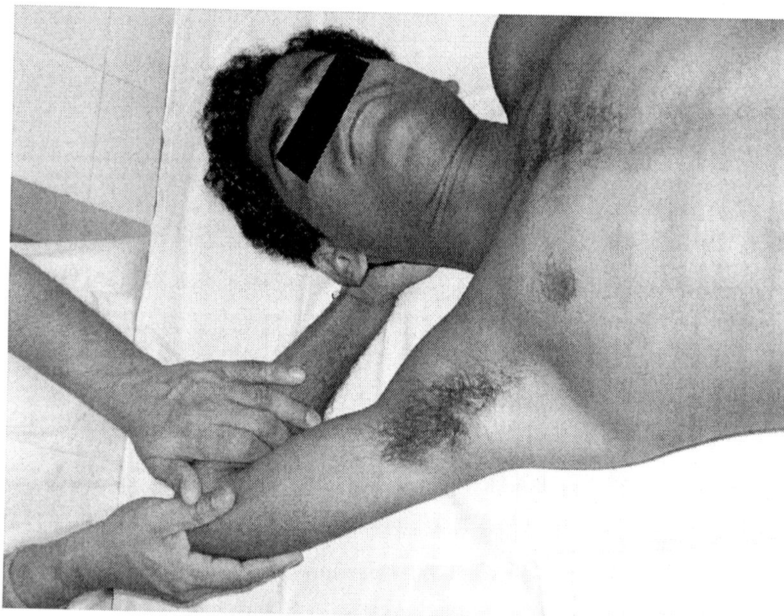

Fig. 7.4: Stretching of teres major

Latissimus Dorsi (Fig. 7.5)

Elevation of the arm through flexion stretches the Latissimus dorsi.

Rhomboids (Fig. 7.6)

Lie towards prone with the hand on the lower back. Therapist tries to put the fingers underneath the medial border of the scapula to stretch the muscle.

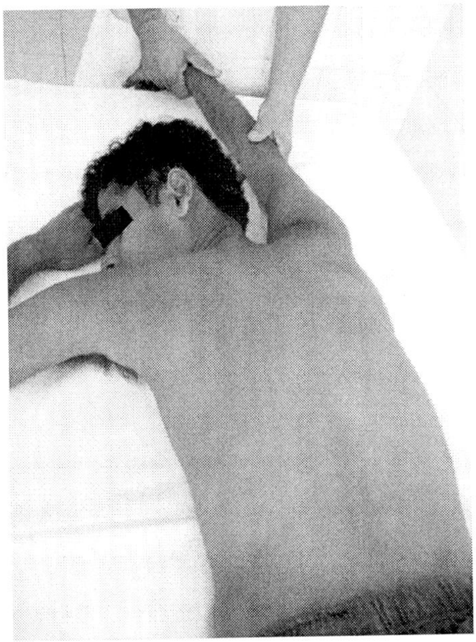

Fig. 7.5: Stretching of latissimus dorsi

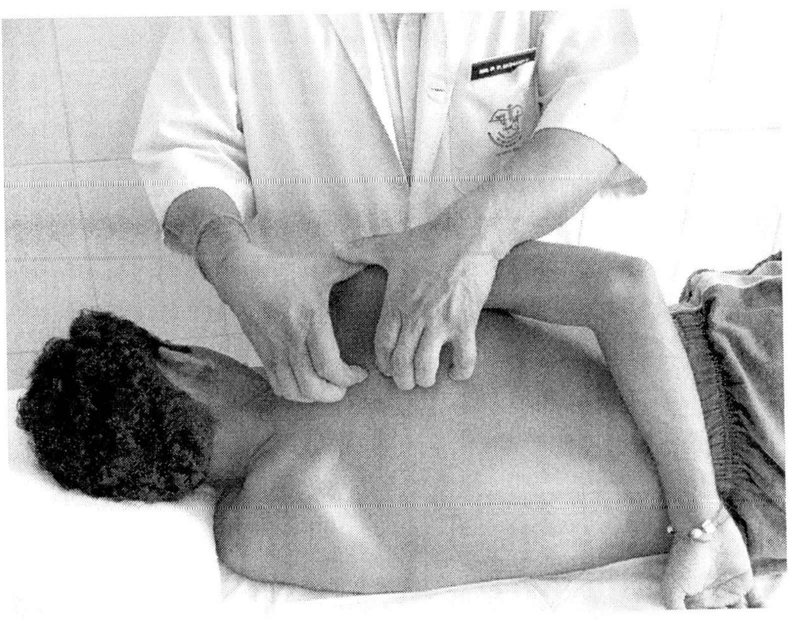

Fig. 7.6: Stretching of rhomboids

Supraspinatus (Fig. 7.7)

Internal rotation of shoulder behind the back stretches the supraspinatus.

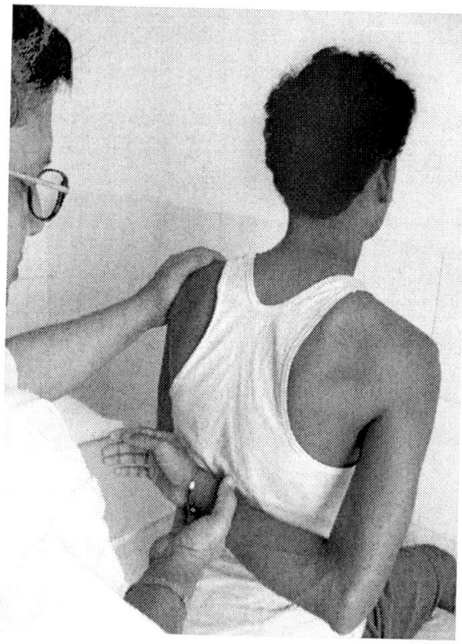

Fig. 7.7: Stretching of supraspinatus

Levator Scapulae (Fig. 7.8)

In sitting position pull the arm, flexed to about 120°, across the forehead with depression of the medial angle of scapula.

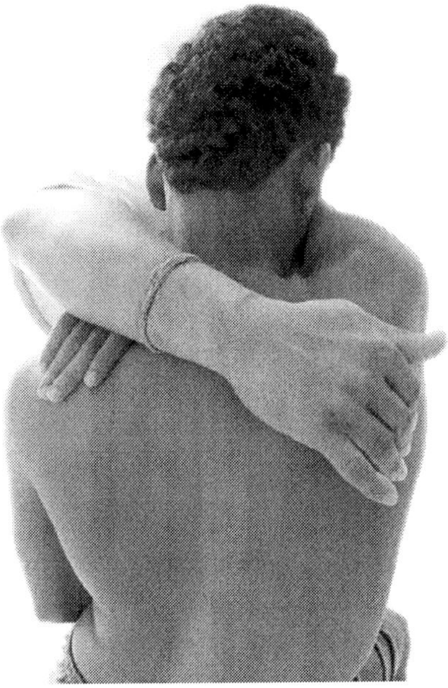

Fig. 7.8: Stretching of levator scapular

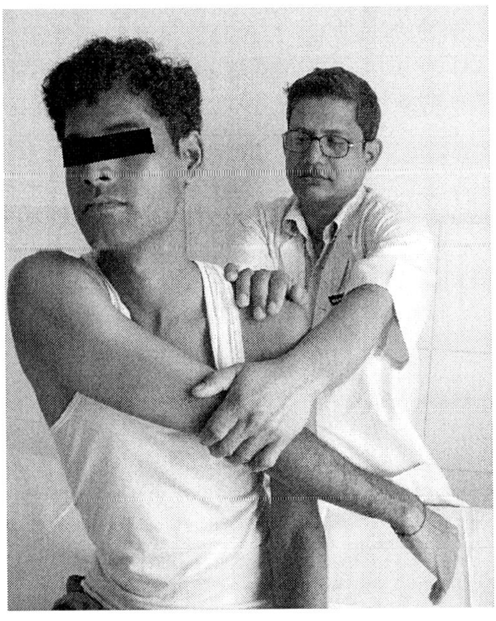

Fig. 7.9: Stretching of infraspinatus

Infraspinatus (Fig. 7.9)

In sitting position pull the arm, flexed to about 60°, across the chest with counter pressure on the back of the opposite shoulder.

BIBLIOGRAPHY

1. Abramson D, Tuck S, et al: Vascular basis for pain due to cold. Arch Phys Med Rehabil, 1996;47:300-05.
2. Antonaci F, et al. Pressure algometry in healthy subjects: Interrex miner variability. Scand J Rehabil Med, 1998;30:3-8.
3. Baker R, Bell GW. The effect of therapeutic modalities on blood flow in the human calf. J Ortho Sports Phys Ther 1991;13:23-7.
4. Barker D, Banks RW. The muscle spindle in A Engle and B Banker, Myology. New York; McGraw - Hill 1986;309-41.
5. Bell WE. Orofacial pains - differential diagnosis, Denedco of Dallas, Dallas, TX 1973.pp.97.
6. Bennett RM. Beyond fibromyalgia: Ideas on etiology and treatment. J Rheum, 1989;16(Suppl 19):185-91.
7. Byl NN, Mc Kenzie, et al. Incisional wound healing: A controlled study of low and high dose ultrasound. J Orthop Sports Phys Ther, 1993;18:619-28.
8. Cameron MH. Physical agents in rehabilitation - from research to practice, 2nd Edition, Saunders, USA: 2003.
9. Carison CR, et al. Reduction of pain and EMG activity in the massager region by Trapezius trigger point injection. Pain, 1993;55: 397-4000.
10. Chaitow L, De Lany J. Clinical application of neuromuscular techniques, in Alternative answers to pain. Churchill Livingstone: 2000.
11. Chaitow L. Modern neuromuscular techniques, New York, Churchill, Livingstone: 1996.
12. Chaitow L. Modern neuromuscular techniques. New York: Churchill Livingstone, 1996,p-114.
13. Chaitow L. Muscle energy techniques, Ed. 2 Churchill Livingstone, Edinburgh: 2001.
14. Chen JT, Chen SM. Phentolamine effect on spontaneous electrical activity of active loci in a myofascial trigger sport of rabbit skeletal muscle. Arch Phys Med Rehabil,1998;79:790-4.
15. Draper DO, Castel JC, Castel D. Rate of temperature increase in human muscle during 1 - Mhz and 3 - Mhz continuous ultrasound. J Orthop Sports Phys Ther, 1995;22:142-50.

16. Draper DO. Anderson C, et al. Immediate and residual changes in dorsiflexion range of motion using an ultrasound heat and stretch routine. J Athl Training, 1988;33:141-4.
17. Draper DO. Do not disregard ultrasound yet - The jury is still out. Phys Ther, 2002;82:190-91.
18. Drapes DO, Schulthies S, et al. Temperature changes in deep muscle of human during ice and ultrasound therapies: an in-vivo study. J Orthop Sports Phys. Ther 1995;21:153-7.
19. Drapes DO, Sunderland S, et al. A comparison of temperature rise in human calf muscle following applications of underwater and topical gel ultrasound. J Orthop Sorts Phys Ther. 1993;17:247-51.
20. Drapper DO. Guidelines to enhance therapeutic ultrasound treatment outcomes. Athletic Therapy Today, 1998;3:7-11.
21. Dyson M, Suckling J. Stimulation of tissue repair by ultrasound: A survey of mechanisms involved. Phys Ther, 1978;64:105.
22. Dyson M. Mechanisms involved in therapeutic ultrasound. Physiother, 1987;73:116-20.
23. Esenyel M, Caglar N. treatment of myofascial pain. Am J Phys Med Rehabil 2000;79:49-52.
24. Esposite CJ, Veal SJ, Farman Ah. Alleviation of myofascial pain with ultrasound therapy. J Prosthet Dent, 1984;51:106-8.
25. Fashbain DA, Goldberg M, et al. Male and Female chronic pain patients categorized by DSM-III, psychiatric diagnostic criteria, Pain, 1986;26:181-97.
26. Fischer AA. Pressure algometry over normal muscles; standard values, validity and reproducibility of pressure threshold. Pain, 30;115-26.
27. Fishcher A. A documentation of myofascial trigger point. Arch Phys Med Rehabil 1998;69:286-91.
28. Forrest G, Rosen C. Ultrasound: Effectiveness of treatment given under water. Arch Phys Med Rehabil, 1989;70;83-5.
29. Fountain F, Gersten JW, Sengu O. Decrease in muscle spasm produced by ultrasound, hot packs and IR. Arch Phys Med Rehabil, 1960;41:293-8.
30. Fricton JR, Kroening R, et al. Myofascial pain syndrome of the head and neck: a review of clinical characteristics of 164 patients. Oral Surg Oral Med Oral Patho, 1985;60;615-23.
31. Gaff - 'Radford SB, Reeves JL, et at. Effects of transcutaneous electrical nerve stimulation on myofascial pain and trigger point sensitivity. Pain 1989;37:1-5.
32. Gam AN, Johanssen F. Ultrasound therapy in musculoskeletal disorders: a metal-analysis. Pain 1995;63:85-91.

33. Gam AW, Warming S. Treatment of myofascial trigger points with ultrasound combined with massage and exercise - a randomized controlled trial Pain, 1998;77:73-9.
34. Gann N. Ultrasound: Current concepts. Clin Mang, 1991;11:64-9.
35. Garvay TA, Marks MR, Wiesel SW. A prospective, randomized double blind evaluation of trigger point injection therapy for low - back pain. Spine, 1989;14:962-4.
36. Gaston J. Measurement of pain: The psychometric properties of the pain-O-meter. A simple inexpensive pain assessment tool that could change health care practices. Journal of Pain and Symptom Management, 1996;12:172-81.
37. Gerecz - Simon E, Tunks E, et al. Measurement of pain threshold in patients with rheumatoid arthritis, osteoarthritis, ankylosing spondylitis and healthy controls. Clin Rheumatol, 1989;8:467-74.
38. Gersten JW. Effects of ultrasound on tendon extensibility. Am J Phys Med. 1955;34;(2):362-9.
39. Graff - Radford SB, Jaeger B, et al. Myofascial pain may present clinically or occipital neuralgia. Neurosurgery 1986;19:610-13.
40. Hanten WP, Olson SL, et al. Effectiveness of a home programme of ischemic pressure followed by sustained stretch for treatment of myofascial trigger points. Phys Thre 2000;88:997-1003.
41. Heuser J, Miledi R. Effects of lanthanum ions on function and structure of frog neuromuscular junction. Proc R Soc Cond B Biol Sci, 1971;179:247-60.
42. Hong C-Z, Simons DG, Statham L. Electromyographic analysis of local twitch responses of human extensor digitorum communis muscle during ischaemic compression over the arm. Arch Phys Med Rehabil 1986;67:680.
43. Hong CZ, Simons DG. Pathophysiology and electrophysiologic mechanisms of myofascial trigger points. Arch Phys Med Rehabil, 1998;79:863-72.
44. Hong CZ, Simons DG. Remote inactivation of myofascial trigger point by inject of trigger point in another muscle. Scand J. Rheumatol 1992;94 (Suppl):24.
45. Hong CZ, Torigoe Y. Electrophysiological characteristics of localized twitch responses in responsive bands of rabbit skeletal muscle fibres. J Musculoskelet pain, 1994;21:17-43.
46. Hong CZ. Persistence of local twitch response with loss of conduction to and from the spinal cord. Arch Phys Med Rehabil, 1994;75:12-6.
47. Hong CZ: Chen YC, et al. Immediate effects of various physical medicine modalities on pain threshold of an active myofascial trigger point. J Musculoskeletal Pain, 1993;1:37-53.

48. Hong CZ: Persistence of local twitch response with loss of conduction to and from the spinal cord. Arch Phys Med Rehabil 1994;75:12-6.
49. Hou CR, et al. Immediate effects of various physical therapeutic modalities on cervical myofascial pain and trigger- point sensitivity. Arch Phys Med Rehabil, 2002;83:1406-14.
50. Howgweg J, A Langereis MJ, et al. Algometry: measuring pain threshold, method and characteristics in healthy subjects. Scand J Rehabil Med. 1992;24:99-103.
51. Hsieh C, Yeung B. Active neck motion measurements with a tape measure J Orthop Phys Ther, 1986;8:88-92.
52. Hsueh TC, et al: The immediate effectiveness of electrical nerve stimulation and electrical muscle stimulation on myofascial trigger points. Am J Phys Med Rehabil 1997;76:47-476.
53. Hubbard Dr, Berkoff GM. Myofascial trigger points show spontaneous needle EMG activity. Spine, 1993;18:1803-07.
54. Hubbard DR. Chronic and recurrent muscle pain. Pathophysiology and treatment, and review of pharmacological studies. J Musculoskeletal pain, 1996;4:123-43.
55. Hunt CC, Jami C, et al. Effects of stimulating the lumbar sympathetic trunk on cat hindlimb muscle spindles. Archieves Italiennes de Biologie, 1982;120:371-84.
56. Huskisson E, Dudly Hart F. Threshold in arthritis. BMJ, 1972;4:193-5.
57. Jaeger N, Reeves JL. Qualification of changes in myofascial trigger point sensitivity with the pressure algometer following passive stretch. Pain, 1986;27;203-10.
58. Jenson K, Anderson HO, et al. Pressure pain threshold in human temporal region: Evaluation of a new pressure algometer. Pain, 1986;25:323-23.
59. Johnson EW. Is there such a thing as myofascial pain, Journal of a back and musculoskeletal rehabilitation, 1997;8:3.
60. Kellgren JH. Observation on referred pain arising from muscle. Clin Sci. 1938;2:175-90.
61. Kelly M. The treatment of fibrositis and allied disorders by local anesthesia. Med J Aust, 1941;1:294-8.
62. Kimura J. Electrodiagnosis in disease of nerve and muscle. Vol. 2; FA Davis, Philadelphia: 1989.
63. Kitchen SS, Partridge J. A review of therapeutic ultrasound. Physiotherapy, 1990;76:593-600.
64. Kosek E, Ekholm J, Nordemar R. A comparison of pressure pain threshold in different tissues and body region. Scand J Rehabil Med, 1993;25:117-23.

65. Kraft GH, Fischer AA: Myofascial Pain - update in diagnosis and treatment. Phys Med Rehabil Clin North Am, 1997;8.
66. Kraybala B, Borg-Stein J, et al. Reduced dizziness and pain with treatment of cervical Myofascial pain. Arch Phys Med Rehabil, 2002;83:540-7.
67. Kuitert J. Ultrasound energy as an adjunct in the management of radiculitis and similar referred pain. Am J Phys Med. 1954:33:61.
68. Lee JC, Lin DT, Hong CZ. The effectiveness of simultaneous thermotherapy with ultrasound and electrotherapy with combined AC and DC current on the immediate pain relief to myofascial trigger point. J Musculoskel Pain 1997;5:81-90.
69. Lehman J, De Lateur BJ, et al. Selective heating effects of ultrasound inhuman beings. Arch Phys Rehabil, 1985;66;331.
70. Lehman J, Lateur BJ, et al. Heating produced by ultrasound in bone and soft tissue. Arch Phys Med Rehabil, 1967;48:397-401.
71. Lehmann JF, Delteur BJ, et al: Therapeutic temperature distribution produced by ultrasound as modified by dosage and volume of tissue exposed. Arch Phys Med Rehabil 1967;47:662-6.
72. Lewit K, simons DG. Myofascial pain: Relief by post-isometric relaxation. Arch Phys Med Rehabil 1984;65;452-6.
73. Lewit K. Manipulative therapy in rehabilitation of the locomotor system, 2nd Ed. Butterworth Heinemann, Oxford: 1991.
74. Lowe J, Honeyman, Lowe G. Ultrasound treatment of trigger points: differences in technique for myofascial pain syndrome and fibromyalgia patients. Medicine du Sud - est 1999;2:12-15.
75. Lundberg G, Gerdle B. Tender point scores and their relations to signs of mobility, symptoms and disability in female home care personnel and the prevalence of fibromyalgia syndrome. J Reheumatol, 2002;29:603-13.
76. Mc Nulty WH, et al: Needle electromyographic evaluation of trigger point response to a psychological stressor. Phychophysiology, 31; 313-6.
77. Mense S, Simons DG, Russell IJ. Muscle Pain: Understanding its nature, diagnosis, and treatment: Lippincott Williams and Wilkins Philadelphia, 2001.
78. Mense S. Referral of muscle pain: new aspects. Am pain Soc J, 1994;3:1-9.
79. Merrick MA, Bernard KD, et al. Identical 3 - MHz ultrasound treatment with different devices produce different intramuscular temperatures. J Orthop Sports Phys Ther, 2003;33:379-85.
80. Merskey H FG. The reliability of the pressure algometer. British Journal of social and Clinical Psyschology, 1964;3:130-6.

81. Nice DA, Riddle DL, et al. Inter-tester reliability of judgments of the presence of trigger points in patients with low back pain. Arch Phys Med Rehabil, 1992;73:893-8.
82. Njoo KH. The occurrence and inter-rater reliability of myofascial trigger point in the quadratus lumborum and gluteus medius: A prospective study in non-specific low back pain patients and controls in general practice. Pain, 1994;58;317-32.
83. Nussbaum EL. Ultrasound to heat or not to heat - that is the question. Phys Ther Rev, 1997;2:59-72.
84. O' Driscoll S, Jayson M. Pain threshold analysis in patients with osteoarthritis of hip. BMJ 1974;3:714-5.
85. Ohraback R, Gale E. Pressure pain threshold, clinical assessment and differential diagnosis: reliability and validity in patients with myogenic pain. Pain, 1989;39:157-69.
86. Ohrbach R, Gale EN: Pressure pain thresholds in normal muscles: reliability, measurement effects and topographical differences. Pain, 1989;37:257-63.
87. Oison SL, O'Connor DP, et al. Tender point sensitivity, ROM and perceived disability in subjects with neck pain. J Orhtop Sports Phys Ther, 2000;30:13-20.
88. Passatore M, Filippi G. On whether there is a direct sympathetic influence on jaw muscle spindles. Brain Research, 1981;225:162-5.
89. Price D, McGrath P, et al. The validation of visual analogue scales as ratio scale measures for chronic and experimental pain. Pain, 1983;17:45-56.
90. Reaves J, Jaeger H, et al. Reliability of pressure algometer as a measure of my orofascial trigger point sensitivity. Pain, 1986;24: 313-21.
91. Reid DC, Cummings GE: Factors in selecting the dosage of ultrasound. Physiother Can, 1973;2:5-9.
92. Revill S, Robinson J, et al. The reliability of a linear analogue for evaluating pain. Anesthesia, 1976;31:1191-8.
93. Robertson VJ, Baker KG. A review of therapeutic ultrasound: effectiveness studies, Phys Ther, 2001;81:1339-50.
94. Robertson VJ, Spurritt D. Electrophysical agents: implication of EDA availability and use in undergraduate clinical placements. Physiotherapy, 1998;84:335-44.
95. Rubin D. Myofascial trigger point syndrome: An approach to management. Arch Phys Med Rehabil 1981;62:107-14.
96. Russell IJ. Neurochemical pathogenesis of fibromyalgia syndrome. J Musculoskel Pain, 1996;4:61-92.

97. Santini M, Ibata Y. The fine structure of thin unmyelinated axons within muscle spindles. Brain Research, 1971;33:289-302.
98. Schwartz RA, et al: Personality characteristic of patients with Myofascial pain - dysfunction syndrome: unresponsiveness to conventional therapy. J Dent Res, 1979;58;1435-9.
99. Scott J, Huskisson EC. Vertical or horizontal analogue scale. Am Rehum Dis. 1979;38:560.
100. Sharav Y, Tzukert A, Refaeli B. Muscle pain index in relation to pain, dysfunction and dizziness associated with the Myofascial pain - Dysfunction syndrome. Oral Surg 1978;46;741-7.
101. Simms RW, Goldernberg DL, et al. Tenderness in 75 anatomic sites: Distinguishing fibromyalgia patients from controls. Arthritis Rheum, 1988;31:182-7.
102. Simons DG, Hong CZ, Simons LC. Prevalence of spontaneous electrical activity at trigger spots and at control sites in rabbit skeletal muscle. J Musculoskel Pain, 1995;3:35-48.
103. Simons DG, Hong CZ: Simons LS: End plate potentials are common to did fiber myofascial trigger points. Am J Phys Med Rehabil 2002;81;212-22.
104. Simons DG, Mense S. Understanding and measurement of muscle tone as related to clinical muscle pain. Pain, 1998;76;1-17.
105. Simons DG, Stolov WC. Microscopic feature and transient contraction of palpable bands in canine muscle. Am J Phys Med, 1976;55:65-88.
106. Simons DG. Clinical and etiological update of myofascial pain from trigger points. J Musculoskel Pain, 1996;4:93-121.
107. Simons DG. Myofascial trigger points: A need for understanding. Arch Phys Med Rehabil 1981;62:97-9.
108. Skootsky SA, Jaeger B, Oye RK. Prevalance of myofascial pain in general internal medicine practice. West J Med, 1989;151:157-60.
109. Sola AE, Rodenberger ML, Gettys BB. Incidence of hypersensitive areas in posterior shoulder muscles. Am J Phys Med, 1995;34:585-90.
110. Stein J, Simons DG. Myofascial pain. Arch Phys Med. Rehabil, 2002;83(Suppl 1):540-7.
111. Takala EP. Pressure pain threshold on upper trapezius and levator scapulae muscles. Scand J Rehabil Med, 1990;22:63-8.
112. Talaat AM, et al. Physical Therpay in the management of Myofascial pain dysfunction syndrome. AM Otol Rhino Laryngol, 1986;95:225.
113. Taylor Robbins C. Continuous ultrasound in the treatment of myofascial trigger point: an opinion. The Journal of Myofascial Therapy, 1994;1:12.

114. Travell J, Rinzler S, et al: Pain and disability of the shoulder and arm; treatment by intramuscular infiltration with procain hydrochloride. JAMA 1942;120:417-22.
115. Travell J, Rinzler SH. The myofascial genesis of pain. Postgrad Med, 1952;11:425-34.
116. Travell J, Simons DG. Myofascial pain and dysfunction: the trigger point manual. Vol. 2 the lower extremities. Baltimore: Williams and Wilkins, 1992.
117. Travell JG, Simons DG. Myofascial pain and dysfunction: The trigger point manual. Baltimore (MD): Williams and Wilkins: 1983;1.
118. Tunks E. Crook J, et al. Tender points in fibromyalgia. Pain, 1988;34: 11-19.
119. Vatine J, Shapira SC, et al. Electronic pressure algometry of deep pain in healthy volunteers. Arch Phys Med Rehabil, 1993;74:526-30.
120. Vecchiet L, Vecchiet J, et al. Referred muscle pain; clinical and pathophysiologic aspects. Curr Rev Pain, 1999;3:489-98.
121. Viitanòn JV, Kokkom L, et al. Neck mobility assessment in ankylosing spondylitis: A clinical study for cervical rotation and lateral flexion. British Journal of Rheumatology, 1998;37:377-81.
122. Weeks VD, Travell J. How to give painless injections AMA Scientific exhibits. Gruna and Stratton, New York, 1957.
123. Wertz RL. Myofascial trigger point therapy and soft tissue pain management. www.drwertzseminars.com.
124. Windt, et al. Ultrasound therapy for musculoskeletal disorders: a systematic review. Pain, 1999;81:257-71.
125. Wolf F, Smythe Ha, et al: The American College of Rhematology 1990 criteria for the classification of fibromyalgia: Report of the multicentre criteria committee Arthritis Rheum, 1990;33:160-72.
126. Wolfe F, Cathey MA. Prevalence of primary and secondary fibrositis. J Rheumator, 1983;10:965-8.
127. Wolfe F, Simons DG, Fricton J. The fibromyalgia and myofascial pain syndromes: A preliminary study of tender points and trigger points in persons with fibromyalgia, myofascial pain syndrome and no disease. J of Rheumatol, 1992;19:944-51.
128. Yunus MB, Mari at, el al: Primary fibromyalgia: clinical study of 50 patients with matched normal controls. Semin Arthritis Rheum. 1981;11:151-71.
129. Zusman M. The ability visual analogue scale as a measure of pain intensity Australian Journal of Physiotherapy 1986;32:244-0.

Chapter

8

Painful Hemiplegic Shoulder

Shoulder pain resulting from hemiplegia is a common clinical consequence of focal cerebral insult resulting from vascular lesion (i.e. Hemorrhagic or ischemic stroke). The incidence of shoulder pain varies between studies with estimates which range from 48 to 84% (Najenson et al. 1971, Poulin de Courval et al.1990). Shoulder pain, by itself, can result in significant disability (Najenson et al. 1971, Poduri 1993) and although it can occur as early as 2 weeks post-stroke, a time of 2–3 months post-stroke is more typical (Poduri 1993), in recent prospective study, Gamble et al (2002) reported that 52/152 (34%) developed shoulder pain following stroke, 28% by 2 weeks and 87% by 2 months, by 6 months the pain had resolved in 80% of patients with first ever stroke, who remained from an original cohort of 416 patients, experienced shoulder pain by month 16. Approximately, half of these patients developed pain between stroke onset and 4 months.

Shoulder pain can negatively affect rehabilitation outcomes as good shoulder function is a prerequisite for succesful transfer, maintaining balance, performing activities of daily living and for effective hand function (Risk et al. 1984). Lo et al. (2005) catalogued the diffrent types of shoulder dysfunction based on both clinical and arthrographic findings and reported that 16% of patients of a cohort of 32 patients with hemiplegic shoulder pain within 1 year of stroke had shoulder hand syndrome, 4% had rotator cuff tears, and 50% suffered from frozen shoulder, 63% patient had single type of dysfunction while 34% had two types.

CAUSES OF HEMIPLEGIC SHOULDER PAIN

Although many etiologies have been proposed for shoulder pain, increasingly it appears to be a consequence of spasticity and sustained hemiplegic posture. Shoulder pain may be more common among patients with neglect following stroke (Kaplan 1995). Possible sources of hemiplegic shoulder pain are impingement of rotator cuff or subacromial bursa, rotator cuff tendonitis, glenohumeral subluxation, adhesive capsulitis, shoulder hand syndrome, spasticity and contracture, etc. Factors most frequently associated with shoulder pain are glenohumeral subluxation (Crossens-sills and Schenkman 1985, Mokowitz et al. 1969, Savage and Robertson 1982, Shai et al. 1984), shoulder contracture or restricted shoulder range of motion (Bloch and Bayer 1978, Brown et al. 1981, Fugl Mayer et al 1975, Crossen -sills and Schenkman 1985, Hakuno et al. 1984, Risk et al.1984) and spasticity particularly of the subscapularis and pectoral muscles (Brown et al. 1981, Caldwell et al 1969, Moskowitz 1969a, 1969b). Other suggested causes of shoulder pain include reflex sympathetic dystrophy (Chu et al. 1981, Davis et al. 1977, Perrigot et al. 1975), or injury to rotator cuff musculotendinous unit (Nejlson et al.1979, Nepomuceno et al 1974). The role of central post-stroke pain in the etiology of shoulder pain is unclear (Walsh 2001).

Shoulder Subluxation

Shoulder subluxation is best defined as changes in the mechanical integrity of the glenohumeral joint causing a palpable gap between the acromion and humeral head. The most reliable clinical measurement of the subacromial space used in clinical research is callipers (Boyd 1992). Glenohumeral joint is multiaxial and has range of motion which exceeds than that of other joints in the body. To achieve this mobility the glenohumeral joint must sacrifice stability. Stability is achieved through the rotator cuff musculotendinous sleeve, which maintains the humeral head in glenoid fossa, while at the same time allowing shoulder mobility. During the initial period following a stroke hemiplegic arm is flaccid or hypotonic. Therefore the shoulder musculatures in particular the rotator cuff musculotendinous sleeve cannot perform the function of maintaining the humeral head in glenoid fossa and there is high risk of shoulder subluxation.

Shoulder subluxation is very common problem in hemiplegic patients. During the initial flaccid stage of hemiplegia the involved extremity must be adequately supported or the weight of the arm will result in shoulder subluxation. Improper positioning in bed, lack of support while the patient is in upright position or pulling on the hemiplegic arm when transferring the patient all contribute to glenohumeral subluxation. Down and lateral subluxation commonly occurs secondary to prolong downward pull on the arm against which hypotonic muscles offer little resistance. The resulting mechanical effect is over-stretching of glenohumeral capsule (especially in superior aspect)and flaccid supraspinatus and deltoid muscles (Basmajin and Bazant 1959, shahani, et al.1981)

Basmajian and Bazant (1959) proposed that in the normal state, subluxation of the humeral head is prevented by upper part of shoulder capsule, coracohumeral ligament provided glenoid fossa is angulated upward. After hemiplegic stroke they hypothetised that upward angulation of scapula would be lost. Calliet (1980) added that in the flaccid stage the scapula assumed depressed and downward rotated position as the paretic serratus anterior and upper part of trapezius no longer supports the scapula. The combination of flaccid supportive musculature (in particular supraspinatus muscle) and a downward rotated scapula was presumed to be predisposing the head of humerus to undergo inferior subluxation relative to glenoid fossa. Prevost, et al. (1987), using 3D X-ray technique, studied movements of scapula and humerus in stroke patients. They studied 50 stroke patients comparing affected and nonaffected shoulder in terms of vertical position of humerus (i.e. degree of subluxation) in relation to scapula. The orientation of the glenoid fossa was also different. However they found that with subluxed shoulder it was facing less downward. There was no significant relationship found between the orientation of the scapula and severity of subluxation. They concluded that scapular orientation was not an important factor in the occurrence of inferior subluxation in hemiplegia (Prevost et al 1987). Culham et al (1995) reported that while patients with low tone had significantly greater subluxation compared to high tone group (0.52 vs 0.21) there was no corelation between the amount of subluxation and scapular abduction angle or the humeral abduction angle. Price et al (2001) compared patients with and without stroke and reported that subluxation in stroke patients was unrelated to scapular resting position. These authors reported that normal scapula tilts downward to greater degree found in other studies.

Pain in Shoulder Subluxation

Shoulder subluxation may be associated with several conditions including: shoulder pain (Crossens-sills and Schenkman 1985, Moskowitz et al. 1969b, Savage and Robertson 1982, Shai et al. 1984, Roy et al. 1994) and frozen shoulder and brachial plexus traction injury (Kingery et al. 1993). It has been assumed that if not corrected, a pattern of traction on flaccid shoulder will result in pain, decreased range of motion and contracture. However, not all patients with subluxed hemiplegic shoulder experience shoulder pain and it remains controversial as to whether it causes hemiplegic shoulder pain (Fitzgerald-Finch and Gibson 1975, Moskowitz et al. 1969b, Sahani, et al. 1981, Bender and Mckenna 2001). Failure to consistently report an association may be due in part failure to examine the contribution of other probable etiological factors concurrently and to account for the chronicity of stroke since there is correlation between early signs of shoulder subluxation and development of pain. Paci et al. (2005) suggested that pain associated with subluxation is probably later after stroke since "fibrous change or injury can occur in connective tissue of ligaments and joint capsule due to incorrect alignment between humerus and scapula". Although several studies have reported an association, others have not confirmed this finding. Heterogenicity of patient characteristics and timing and method of assessment (radiological vs clinical examination) may account for the lack of consistency of findings.

Conclusion

Shoulder subluxation occurs early on hemiplegic arm due to flaccid supporting shoulder musculature and is not result of downward scapular rotation.

Shoulder subluxation may be cause of shoulder pain. However, patients with subluxation do not necessarily experience pain and not all cases of hemiplegic shoulder pain suffer from subluxation.

Although it has not been established that shoulder subluxation is the primary cause of hemiplegic shoulder pain it would still seem prudent to take care early on with the hemiplegic upper extremity to avoid subluxation.

Spasticity

Abnormal muscle tone, including spasticity may be directly related to hemiplegic shoulder pain. Spasticity is defined as velocity dependent increase in resistance to passive stretch of muscles accompanied by hyperactive muscle stretch reflexes and often associated with clasp knife phenomenon. Spasticity is one component of UMN syndrome and is the inevitable accompaniment of hemiplegia and an incomplete motor recovery. Under normal circumstances a delicate balance exists between facilitating and inhibiting influences upon both alpha and gamma motor neurons which together maintain appropriate control of skeletal muscle length and strength of contraction at the spinal cord level. After a stroke input from one or more of the supraspinal suppressor areas will decrease or stop entirely. The balance of control over the muscle tips in favour of facilitation and spasticity results only if there is loss of input from both pyramidal and extrapyramidal motor systems. Spasticity presents as increased tone and reflexes on the involved side of body. Van Ouwenaller et al. (1986) looked at various factors in 219 patients followed for one year after stroke and identified much higher incidence of shoulder pain in spastic (85%) than in flaccid (18%) hemiplegics. They identified spasticity as prime factor and the one most frequently encountered in the genesis of shoulder pain in the hemiplegic patients. They were unsure of the etiology of subsequent shoulder pain. Poulin de Courval et al. (1990) examined 94 hemiplegic patients involved in rehabilitation program after stroke and reported that subjects with shoulder pain had significantly more spasticity of the affected limb than those without pain. In contrast Bohannon et al. (1986) conducted a statistical analysis of 50 consecutive hemiplegic patients (36 with shoulder pain) and asserted that spasticity was unrelated to pain. Joynt (1920) also supported this finding after examining 67 patients with shoulder problems following stroke. Nevertheless, evidence for spasticity in particular hypertonic muscle imbalance, as cause of hemiplegic shoulder pain is growing.

Hemiplegia following stroke is characterized by typical posturing reflecting hypertonic muscle patterns, flexor tone predominates in the hemiplegic upper extremity and results in scapular retraction and depesssion as well as internal rotation and adduction of the shoulder. This posture is consequence of ablation of higher centers and subsequent release of motor groups from pyramidal and extrapyramidal control. In stroke recovery this synergy pattern is inevitable where recovery is incomplete, one consequence of this development of spastic muscle imbalance about shoulder joint.

Clinically the internal rotators of the shoulder predominate after a stroke involving that arm and external rotation is one of the last areas of shoulder function to recover. Hence during recovery motor units are not appropriately recruited or turned off, the result is simultaneous cocontraction of agonist and antagonist muscles. A shortened agonist in the synergy pattern becomes stronger and the constant tension of agonist can become painful. Stretching of these tightened spastic muscles causes more pain. Shortened muscle inhibits movement, reduces range of motion and prevents other movement. Especially at the shoulder where the external rotation of humerus is necessary for arm abduction greater than 90 degrees. Muscles that contribute to spastic internal rotation/ adduction of shoulder include the subscapularis, pectoralis major, teres major and latissimus dorsi muscles. However, subscapularis and pectoralis major muscles have been implicated as most often being spastic leading to muscle imbalance.

The subscapularis muscle originates on the undersurface of scapula and inserts on lesser tuberosity of the humerus as well as the capsule of the shoulder joint. It is a major internal rotator of the shoulder (Hollinshed and Jenkins 1981). The subscapularis muscle also participates in arm abduction and extension from flexed position (Cole and Tobis 1990). In normal individuals nerve impulses to the subscapularis muscle are inhibited during arm abduction, the muscle then relaxes and allows the humerus to rotate externally thus prevents impingement of greater tuberosity on acromion (Codman1934). As part of typical flexor synergy pattern in spastic hemiplegics internal rotators including the subscapularis muscle are tonically active; this limits shoulder abduction, flexion and external rotation.

Bohannon et al 1986 found limitation of shoulder external rotation of the hemiplegic shoulder was the factor which most correlated with hemiplegic shoulder pain. Zorowitz et al. (1996) also found that limitation in shoulder external rotation correlated strongly with pain. Hecht (1995) specifically linked this problem to subscapularis muscle when he noted "the subscapularis muscle is the primary cause of shoulder pain in spastic hemiplegia where external rotation is most limited although other muscles may contribute to spasticity, pain and functional contracture, the subscapularis is the keystone of the abnormal synergy pattern.

The pectoralis major muscle serves to forward flexion, adduction and internally rotates the arm. Hecht (1995) has reported on subset of hemiplegic patients with greater limitation in abduction (and flexion) than on external rotation. In these patients a spastic pectoralis muscle appears to be problematic. This disorder is characterized by motion being most limited and pain produced on abduction. A tight band of spastic muscle can be palpated in the anterior axillary fold (Hecth1995). It is also noteworthy that pectoralis major muscle is a synergist of subscapularis muscle.

Frozen Shoulder

A frozen shoulder is characterized clinically by limitation in range of movement, with pattern of restriction. This condition is frequently identified as source of pain in spastic hemiplegic shoulder (Bohannon, et al. 1986, Eto et al. 1980, Fugl mayor et al 1975, Grossen-sills and schenkman 1985, Hakuno et al. 1984, Risk et al. 1984). Hakunoetal et al. 1984 studied both the affected and sound sides shoulder of 77 patients with hemiplegia due to stroke by positive contrast arthography and found significantly higher rate (54.6%) adhesive capsulitis in the paralyzed shoulder than in the non-paralyzed side (32.5%). Loss of movements both in flaccid and spastic stages result in adaptive shortening of the capsule, where it is loose. Adhesion and shortening of inferior capsular fold limits shoulder abduction, shortening of anterior joint capsule limits shoulder external rotation and extension; and that of posterior capsule restricts internal rotation and flexion. To prevent adhesive capsulitis relaxed passive movements with normal arthrokinematics should be given.

In summary while shoulder subluxation is not always associated with shoulder pain. The problem of hemiplegic shoulder pain appears to be due to combination of spastic muscle imbalance and frozen contracted shoulder. However, overaggressive stretching of shoulder through an aggressive stretching program may simply aggravate the pain as it does not address the issue of spastic muscle imbalance.

Conclusion

There is an association between spasticity and the development of hemiplegic shoulder pain. Spasticity and subsequent frozen shoulder are most likely causes of hemiplegic shoulder pain. Spasticity and hemiplegic shoulder pain are related.

ROTATOR CUFF DISORDERS

Because shoulder pain is so often associated with rotator cuff disorders in nonstroke population it should not be surprising that it would be seen as potentially common cause of hemiplegic shoulder pain. However, Risk et al. (1984) failed to demonstrate any evidence of rotator cuff tears on arthrography in 30 patients with hemiplegic shoulder pain. A similar study (Nepomuceno and Miller 1974) reported a 33% incidence of rotator cuff tear in painful shoulders after strokes. Najenson et al. (1971) reported that 13 of 32 (40%) patients with severe paralysis of upper extremity were found to have rupture of rotator cuff ligaments based on arthographic findings. Partial tears of rotator cuff musculature are common and it is always difficult determining whether they were present premorbidly even in previously asymptomatic patients. Joynt (1992) diagnosed 67 stroke patients as having hemiplegic shoulder pain. 28 patients received a subacromial injection of lidocaine; approximately half obtained moderate or marked relief of pain and improved range of motion. However, this provides only indirect evidence of rotator cuff disorders as a possible cause of hemiplegic shoulder pain. Generally, hemiplegic shoulder pain is not commonly associated with rotator cuff disorder.

Development of painful hemiplegic shoulder is associated with severe strokes and poorer functional outcome. Wankylin et al. 1996 studied 108 post-stroke patients over the age of 60 and found 63.8% of all patients developed shoulder pain associated with reduced shoulder shrug and reduced pinch grip. Patients who required assistance for transfer were more likely to suffer with shoulder pain. Aras et al. (2004) found 54 out of 85 stroke patients having shoulder pain. Shoulder pain was reported more frequently among patients with reflex sympathetic dystrophy, sublaxation, limitation of shoulder external rotation and flexion and poor shoulder functional level.

MANAGEMENT OF PAINFUL HEMIPLEGIC SHOULDER

Once the condition has devloped, it is difficult and response to treatment is frequently unsatisfactory (Risk, et al 1984). The best treatment approach has not been definitely established in part due to uncertainty in etiology of the pain. As a result a wide variety of treatments have been used, with varying degrees of success (Snels et al. 2002). Ideally measures should be taken immediately following stroke to minimize the potential risk for the devlopment of pain. Early passive shoulder range of motion and supporting and protecting the involved shoulder, in the initial flaccid stage are regarded as important steps to reduce the devlopment of shoulder pain.

Positioning

The muscles around shoulder are often paralyzed, initially with flaccid tone and later with spasticity. Careful positioning of shoulder helps to minimize subluxation and later contractures as well as possibly promote recovery while poor positioning may adversly affect symmetry balance and body image as cited by Gilimore et al. (2004). Davis (2000) suggested that shoulder pain can be prevented through correct and careful positioning. Bender and McKenna (2001) have noted that primary goal of stroke rehabilitation is to prevent devlopment of hypertonicity (Jhonstone 1992) and to discourage inefficient patterns. Bobath (1990), Bender and Mckenna (2001) noted that the recommended position for the upper limb is toward abduction, external rotation and flexion of the shoulder, however from Carr and Kenny (1992) review, Bender and Mckenna cited that most popular theories failed to yield consensus for exact degrees of positioning.

Dean et al. (2000) found no significant difference between the groups in level of pain, and active and passive range of motion after receiving active training of reaching and manipulation tasks (both the control and experimental groups) and positioning to the affected side (experimental group). Adalo, et al. (2005) found positioning the shoulder in maximal external rotation position (experimental group) significantly reduced development of contracture as compared with the control group who received only shoulder exercises in a RCT of 30 patients.

There is consensus (level 3) opinion that proper positioning of the hemiplegic shoulder helps to prevent subluxation. However, there is conflicting (level 4) evidence that prolonged positioning does not influence active and passive range of motion or level of pain. Further research is needed before conclusions regarding positioning of the hemiplegic shoulder can be made.

Arm Slings

In 1950 and 1960, arm slings (orthopedic sling) (Fig. 8.1) were used during the initial stage following stroke to support the affected arm. However, they are controversial and they can have disadvantages that they increase flexor synergies, inhibit arm swing; contribute to contracture formation and decrease body image causing the patient to further avoid using that arm. However, a sling remains the best method of supporting the flaccid hemiplegic arm while the patient is standing or transferring.

Rolyan hemi arm sling (Fig. 8.2) (Rolyan Smith and Nephew, Inc., Menomonee Falls, WI) has a humeral cuff and a figure of eight suspension. It provides moderate support to the humerus and allows the elbow to be extended. The arm is free to be moved and used for support.

Shoulder saddle sling (Fig. 8.3) (Fred Sammons. Inc. Brookfield, II) has a forearm cuff and a shoulder saddle

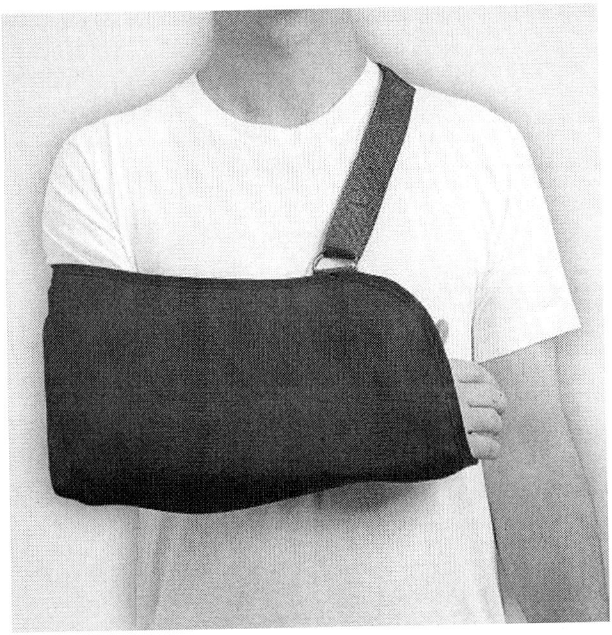

Fig. 8.1: Arm sling

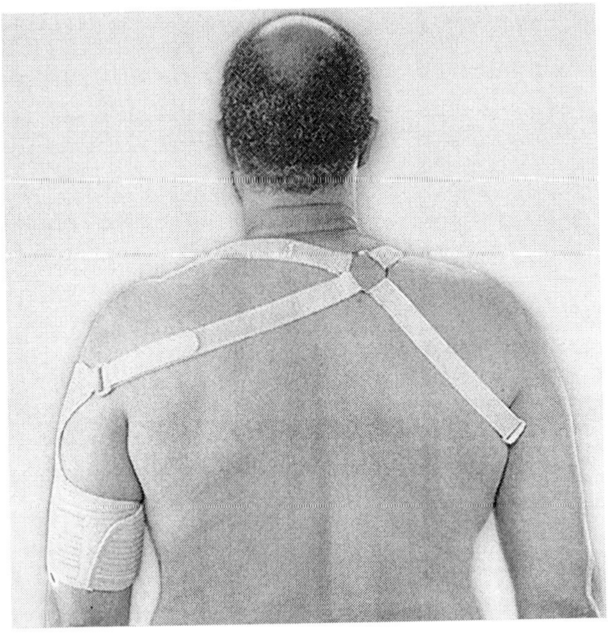

Fig. 8.2: Roylan sling

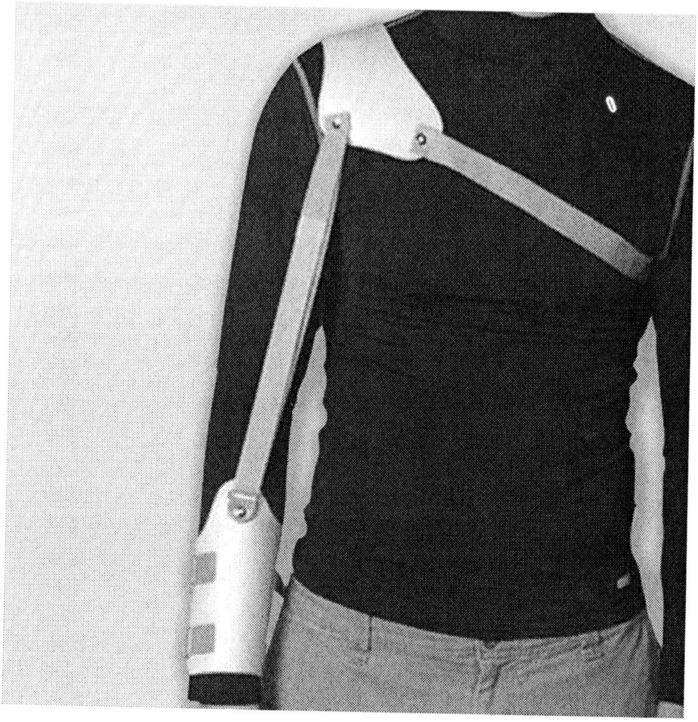

Fig. 8.3: Saddle sling

suspension. It provides maximum support to the entire arm and prevents the arm from banging around during functional activities. The sling is excellent for flaccid limb with pain. It allows moderate humeral and elbow movement.

Axillary strap (All Orthopedic appliances, Inc. Miami, FL) elevates the scapula to neutral alignment and provides minimal inferior support for the humerus. Superior joint capsule and coracohumeral ligament prevent inferior subluxation of the humeral head provided glenoid fossa is angulated upward. It may compress the neurovascular structures in the axilla.

Ada et al (2005) conducted a systematic cochrane review, which included only four RCTs (Ancliffe et al 1992, Griffin, et al. 2003 (unpublished data), Hanger et al. 2000 and Hurd et al 1974) evaluating the benefit of shoulder slings and supports and concluded that there is insufficient evidence that these devices reduce or prevent shoulder subluxation following a stroke.

Hurd et al. 1974 studied 14 patients with or without sling and assessed after 2–3 weeks and 3–7 months post stroke. Of the 7 patients without slings, 5 had no pain, while 2 had little pain; whereas of the 7 patients with slings, 6 had little pain, while 1 had no pain. Moodie et al. 1986 studied 10 patients by taking series of X-rays of the affected and unaffected shoulders and suggested that sling, trough and lap tray reduced the mean subluxation to within 0.56 cm of the normal control while roll and hook tended to under-correct the subluxation. Williams et al. studied 26 patients by taking of X-rays of the subluxed shoulders with and without two different supports-the Bobath shoulder roll and Henderson shoulder sling and found no significant difference in reduction of inferior suluxation between two types of support, however there was significant difference in measurement with and without the support. Brooke et al. (1991) found better correction of vertical as well as the horizontal displacements by Harris hemi-sling than Bobath sling. Zorowitz et al. (1995) found single strap hemisling corrected vertical displacement, Rolyan humeral cuff sling and Bobath roll significantly reduced vertical displacement, Rolyan humeral cuff sling significantly decreased the total subluxation asymmetry, Bobath roll and Cavaller support produced a significant lateral displacement of the humeral head of the affected shoulder compared with unaffected shoulder.

As the tone returns to the shoulder muscles, the risk of shoulder subluxation decreases and sling can be then withdrawn. Sling tends to hold the limb in poor position which may accentuate an adduction and internal rotation posture and may contribute to shortening of tonically active muscles. In the absence of empirical evidence of their efficiency many devices are available and in common use including variety of slings and lap boards.

Conclusion

There is limited (level 2) evidence that shoulder sling prevents subluxation associated with hemiplegic shoulder pain, although there is also limited (level 2) evidence that one device or method is no better than other.

Strapping

Strapping the hemiplegic shoulder is used as a method to prevent or reduce the severity of shoulder subluxation and many provide some sensory stimulation. There are three different forms of strapping the hemiplegic shoulder which have been described previously:

Ancliff (1992) used 5 cm wide light weight adhesive tapes; the first length of tape was applied to the shoulder half way along the length of the clavicle, continued across the deltoid muscle in diagonal relation, the tape was terminated approximately one quarter of the way along the spine of scapula. A second length of tape was applied in same direction as the first but 2 cm below. A small length tape was applied over the shoulder to secure the ends.

The findings suggested that strapping group experienced a significantly longer pain free period than without strapping group, however all the patients in strapping group eventually experienced pain, the longest pain free period was 25 days.

Morine and Bravo (1997) used a 10 cm wide elastoplast sports tape (Fig. 8.6). The two main supporting tapes were applied first; both were applied using lifting action starting 5 cm above the elbow and moving up the arm front and back crossing at the top of the shoulder. The posterior arm tape was then anchored down past the clavicle whereas the tape from the anterior aspect of the arm came across the shoulder and down past the spine of scapula. They were both supported at the lower end by a short tape to prevent them peeling off.

Hanger et al. (2000) (Fig. 8.4) found no significant improvement in pain, range of motion and functional outcome measures between experimental group, who received strapping

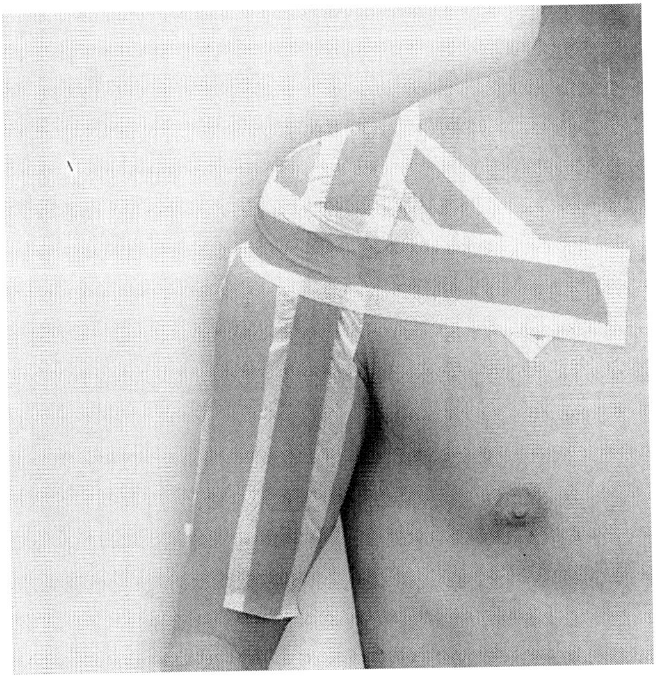

Fig. 8.4: Strapping by Hanger (2000)

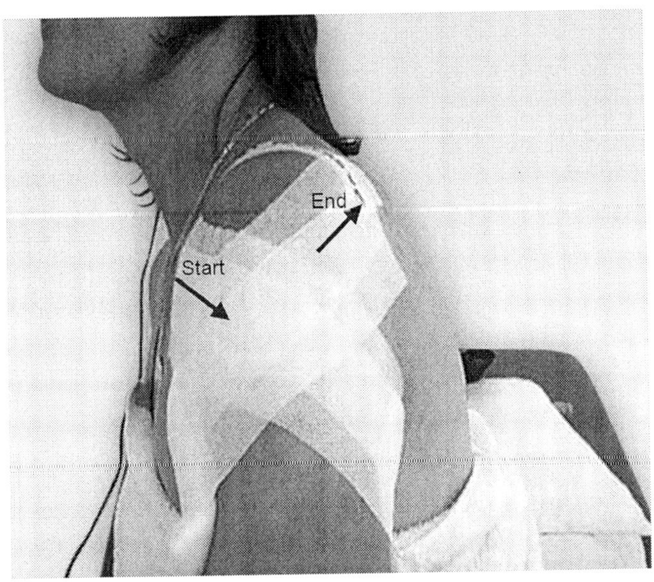

Fig. 8.5: Strapping by Griffin and Bernhardt (2006)

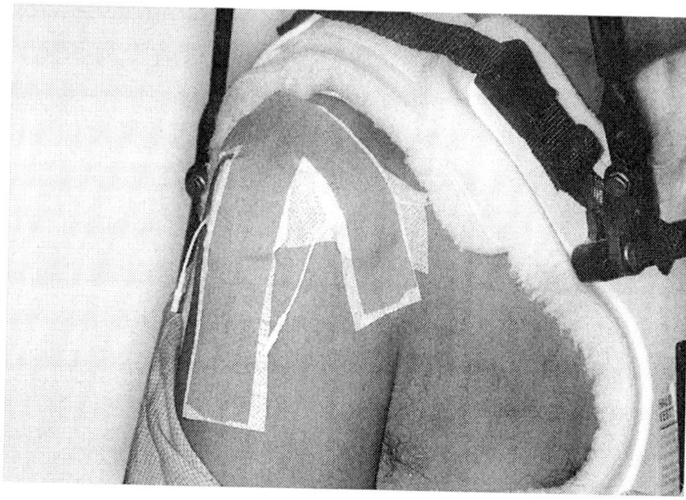

Fig. 8.6: Strapping by Morin and Bravo

for 6 weeks, and the control group, who received only therapy in a RCT of 98 patients. But there was a trend for less pain and improved upper limb functions in the strapping group.

Griffin and Bernhardt (2006) (Fig. 8.5) studied 33 patients for 4 weeks by applying therapeutic shoulder strapping, Sham shoulder strapping and no strapping in a RCT and found therapeutic shoulder strapping group reported 26 pain free days, compared to 19 pain free days for sham shoulder strapping group and 16 days for the control group.

Conclusion

There is conflicting (level 4) evidence that strapping the hemiplegic shoulder reduces the development of pain. There is moderate (level 1b) evidence that strapping does not improve upper limb function or range of motion. Strapping the hemiplegic shoulder does not appear to imprve upper limb function, but may reduce pain.

Active Therpy

The association of spasticity, muscle imbalance and frozen shoulder pain suggest that a therapeutic approach designed to improve range of motion of the hemiplegic shoulder will improve pain.

Inaba, et al (1972) found no significant diffrences in the outcomes of patient who received ROM exercises and positioning, ROM and ultrasound or ROM and mock ultrasound in a RCT of 33 patients. Kumar et al. (1990) found that overhead pullies caused dramatically higher level of shoulder pain than more restrained ROM exercises. Although there were no statistically significant diffrences in change scores between the control and the experimental group. Partridge et al. (1990) found that treatments using Bobath therapy resulted in significantly less pain than cryotherapy. Poduri et al. (1993) reported patients receiving drug therapy experienced pain relief, flexion, abduction and functional recovery to a greater extent than those received only therapy. Lynch et al. (2005) reported a trend towards improvement in the area of shoulder joint stability associated with continuous passive motion using the orthologic static stretches was not only ineffective in reducing loss of range of motion into external rotation but was also associated with increasing levels of pain (Gustafson and Mckenna 2006); counter to previous research subjects in this study continued to improve functionally despite a loss of range of motion and increasing pain reported by subjects in the treatment group.

The general messsage that emerges from these studies is that an active ROM exercises approach is preferable to more passive modalities; but an over aggressive approach (i.e. overhead pulleys) resulted in a very high incidence of hemiplegic shoulder pain when compared to a gentler approach. Adding ultrasound treatment is not helpful while NSAIDs may be helpful.

Conclusion

There is moderate (level 1b) evidence that agresssive range of motion therapies using overhead pullies result in incrased rates of shoulder pain.

There is moderate (level 1b) evidence that Bobath therapy for the hemiplegic shoulder is associated with greater pain reduction than passive cryotherapy (application of local cold therapy).

There is moderate (level 1b) evidence that gentle exercises to improve range of motion is the preferred approach. There is moderate (level 1b) evidence that adding ultrasound therapy to range of motion exercises does not change outcomes.

There is limited (level 2) evidence that providing an oral non-steroidal anti-inflammatory drug leads to less pain, improved range of motion and improved functional recovery in stroke patients with shoulder pain receiving occupational therapy.

There is moderate (level 1b) evidence that static positional stretches performed daily during rehabilitation are associated with increasing pain and decreasing range of motion.

Injections

Corticosteroid and local anesthetic injections are commonly used for shoulder pain in particular rotator cuff tendinopathies. It is not surprising that there would be interest in this mode of treatment in hemiplegic shoulder pain. Joynt (1992) in a retrospective study found 50% of 28 patients who received subacromial injection of 1% lidocaine obtained moderate to marked pain relief and improvement in ROM. Dekker et al. (1997) found intra-articular injections of triamcinolone acetonide demonstrated a significant reduction in pain with highly significant effect in 5 of the 9 patients. One RCT (Snels et al 2000) failed to show the benefit of corticosteroid injections. There is insufficient evidence to recommend this mode of treatment and one trial casting doubt on its efficacy. There is moderate (level 1b) evidence based on one good RCT that corticosteroid injections do not improve shoulder pain or range of motion in patients with hemiplegia. Corticosteroid injections do not improve hemiplegic shoulder pain or range of motion.

Functional Electrical Stimulation

As cited by Gresham et al (1995) the US AHCPR post-stroke rehabilitation guidelines defines FES as bursts of electrical stimulation applied to the nerves or muscles affected by stroke with goal of strengthening muscle contraction and improving motor control. The supraspinatus and posterior deltoid muscles are most likely to be treated as they are important muscles in maintaining the correct alignment of the glenohumeral joint (Paci et al 2005). Theoretically FES should help to compensate or facilitate flaccid shoulder muscles which in turn should reduce the risk of shoulder subluxation. The ideal intensity of treatment is thought to be of 6 hours daily, five days a week for 6 weeks. FES is performed at frequencies of between 35–50 Hz (Paci et al 2005).

Price and Pandyan (2001) conducted a systematic review of all forms of electrical stimulation used in the prevention and treatment of post-stroke shoulder pain. There was evidence that FES in addition to conventional therapy improves function but is not superior for preventing pain. Ada and Foong-chomcheay (2002) also conducted a meta-analysis to examine the effect of electrical stimulation on shoulder subluxation following stroke. This review included the results from 6 RCTs (Baker and Parker 1986, Faghri, et al 1994, Kobayashi et al 1999, Linn et al 1999, Wang et al 2000) and the results suggest that early treatment following stroke helps to prevent development of hemiplegic shoulder while later treatment helps to reduce pain in addition to conventional therapy.

Most of the RCTs (Faghri, et al. 1994, Chantraine, et al. 1999, Yu et al. 2001, Renzenbrink and Ijerman 2004, Yu, et al. 2004, Chaeet al. 2005) reviewed reported a benefit associated with FES/ES treatment, although there was variability in the outcomes assessed range of motion, muscle tone, EMG activity, shoulder subluxation, shoulder pain and muscle function. The results suggest that FES can reduce pain in the affected shoulder and also improve upper extremity function. Percutaneously placed devices may improve treatment compliance, however, results from largest and most methodologically rigorous trials (Church et al 2006) suggest that FES treatment might actually be associated with harm and may worsen arm function especially among those with severe paresis. The authors proposed several mechanisms to potentially explain the findings including overuse and overstimulation of the affected arm and possibility that stimulation interfered with motor re-learning processes, influencing and impending upper limb recovery even after treatment ceased. These authors did not evaluate the benefit of FES with respect to shoulder subluxation and spasticity while noting that there is evidence that FES treatment has been shown to improve these parameters.

Conclusion

There is conflicting (level 4) evidence that functional electrical stimulation reduces pain, improves function and reduces subluxation following stroke. Functional electrical stimulation may not help with recovery of hemiplegic shoulder.

Surgery

Surgery to reverse muscle imbalance could potentially relieve hemiplegic shoulder pain that develops due to spastic muscle imbalance. There is limited (level 2) evidence that surgically resecting the subscapularis and pectoralis muscle tendon improves pain and range of motion in stroke patients with painful hemiplegic shoulder. Further research is needed to confirm these findings.

Motor Blocks

Subscapularis spasticity is characterized by limitation of shoulder external rotation range of motion with pain. Pectoralis muscle spasticity is characterized by limitation of abduction range and pain. This appears to correlate well with hemiplegic shoulder pain that is now thought to be consequence of spastic muscle imbalance about the shoulder in many cases. Motor blocks for spastic muscle imbalance offers the ability to redress that imbalance and relieve hemiplegic shoulder pain.

Studies (Hecht 1992 and 1995, Bhakta, et al. 1996, Yelnik, et al. 2006, Marco et al. 2007) showed that there is improvement in ROM, relief of pain following nerve blocks in cases of muscle imbalance in hemiplegic shoulder.

Conclusion

There is moderate (level 1 b) evidence that motor blocks of the subscapular muscle reduces spastic shoulder pain and improves passive range of motion of hemiplegic shoulder.

There is conflicting (level 4) evidence that motor blocks of the pectoralis major muscle reduces spastic shoulder pain or improves passive range of motion of the hemiplegic shoulder. Deinnervation of the subscapularis muscle may reduce shoulder pain and improve passive range of motion, more so than deinnervation of the pectoralis major muscle.

MISCELLANEOUS TREATMENT

Aromatherapy has shown to help reduce pain and anxiety associated with chronic pain conditions (Buckle 1999). The use of aromatherapy plus acupressure in the treatment of hemiplegic shoulder pain has been investigated in a single RCT (Shin and Lee 2007). The authors speculated that the improvement in shoulder pain might result from an enhancement of the parasympathetic response through the effects of smell and touch that encourage relaxation. Relaxation has been shown previously to alter the perception of pain.

Conclusion

There is a moderate (level 1b) evidence that aromatherapy combined with acupressure can reduce pain associated with painful hemiplegic shoulder.

Summary of the Management of the Painful Hemiplegic Shoulder

Despite the high prevalence of patients suffering from painful hemiplegic shoulders the evidence for effective treatment is underwhelming, there is strong (level 1a) evidence supporting functional electrical stimulation and moderate (level 1b) evidence that overaggressive therapies using pullies substantially increases pain when compared to gentle range of motion therapy approaches. There is insufficiant evidence that positioning of the shoulder, shoulder strapping, local corticosteroids injections and adding local ultrasound therapy do not prevent subluxation, decrease pain or increase functionally.

There have been no RCTs conducted on the use of slings; motor blocks for spastic muscle imbalance or providing NSAIDs medication prior to therapy although there is limited (level 2) evidence of a benefit for all three of these treatment approaches.

There is consensus (level 3) opinion that prevention and avoidance of overaggressive therapy is important. Those individuals caring for the the stroke patients particularly early on, should be aware of the potential for shoulder injury. The shoulder should be carefully positioned and supported against gravity while sitting or standing. Range of motion exercises should not carry the shoulder beyond 90 degrees of flexion and abduction unless there is upward rotation of the scapula and external rotation of the humeral head (Gresham et al. 1995)

SHOULDER-HAND SYNDROME

Shoulder-hand syndrome also known as reflex sympathetic dystrophy and complex regional pain syndrome (type 1) is characterized by numerous peripheral and central nervous system changes. Peripheral changes include vasomotor tone with associated pain and swelling, exquisite tenderness or hyperesthesia, protective immobility, trophic skin changes and vasomotor instability of the involved upper extremity. Central changes include a disruption of sensory cortical processing disinhibition of the motor cortex and disrupted body schema (Moseley et al 2004), Iwata et al (2002) emperically described 3 stages of RSD.

Stage I

Persistent pain, described as burning or aching and aggravated by movement. There is edematous, warm and hyperesthetic extremity.

Stage II

Early trophic changes of the skin, muscle atrophy, vasospasm with hyperhidrosis.

Stage III

Soft tissue dystrophy, frozen shoulder, pain and vasomotor changes.

Shoulder hand syndrome generally presents initially with pain in the shoulder followed by painful, edematous hand and wrist. There is frequently decreased range of motoin at the shoulder and hand while the elbow joint is spared (Davis et al 1997). Passive flexion of the wrist, MCP and PIP joints are painful and limited due to edema over the dorsum of the fingers. As time progresses the extensor tendons become elevated and the collateral ligament shorten. If untreated, it has long been thought that shoulder hand syndrome eventually progresses to a dry cold bluish and atrophied hand.

Shoulder hand syndrome is often regarded as a form of sympathetically mediated pain involving the hemiplegic upper extremity. The relationship between sympathetic nervous system and pain remains hypothetical and has yet to be proven. Shoulder hand syndrome develops in about one in four hemiplegics. It is associated with involvement of the premotor region and spasticity in the involved upper extremity. Diagnosis can be made clinically with metacarpophalangeal joint tenderness to compression is the most consistent sign. While recovery is largely spontaneous condition; that persist for more than 6 months are often difficult to treat.

Pathophysiology

Shoulder hand syndrome has been associated with lesions of premotor area of the brain. The etiology of the shoulder hand syndrome is unknown. The sympathetic nervous system has often been implicated largely because of the associated vasomotor changes. Theoretical peripheral and central etiologies have been proposed—peripheral etiological theories postulate a role of trauma to the peripheral nerves. One of these theories postulates ephaptic conduction between efferent sympathetic nerves and afferent somatic nerves with the later depolarization being perceived as pain. Numerous central etiological theories have been proposed; for instance it has been postulated that there is disruption of the autonomic nervous control from higher CNS center, which directly affects the intermural pool of the spinal cord leading to decreased inhibition of the sympathetic neurons of the lateral horn. Pain either from contractures or shoulder subluxation may stimulate the internuncial pool of the spinal cord resulting in abnormal spinal response. A link between abnormal sympathetic nervous system and pain has also been postulated but never proven.

Geurts et al (2000) systemically reviewed the etiology and treatments of post-stroke hand edema and shoulder hand syndrome. The authors identified 5 etiological theories and 6 therapeutic studies. The authors evaluated the studies based on 11 methodological criteria and by standardized effect sizes. Based on their systematic review of the literature, the authors concluded that the shoulder was involved in only half the cases although all of these cases were characterized by painful swelling of the wrist and hand, thereby suggesting a wrist hand syndrome in half the cases. Furthermore, they have noted that hand edema is not lymphedema and that shoulder hand syndrome usually coincided with increased arterial blood flow. Iwata et al. (2002) suggested that SHS might be due to paresis following stroke, mediated by disruption of homeostasis and the balance between intracellular and extracellular fluid. There possible mechanisms include: i) an increase in capillary blood pressure, caused by a decrease in peripheral venous return and lymph flow ii) a drop in the colloidal osmotic pressure in the early stages of stroke due to an acute phase response; iii) enhanced permeability of capillary walls which may result from synovial inflammation, brought about by rough management of the affected arm and hand.

Davis, et al. (1977) found 12.5% (68/540), Tapperman, et al. (1984) found 25% (21/85), Van Ouwenaller et al. (1986) found 23% in 219 hemiplegics, Kondo et al. found 18.5% (15/81) for patients receiving the protocol to prevent RSD and 32.4% (23/71) among the patients who did not receive it, Gokkaya et al. (2006) found 30.5% (29/95) incidence of RSD in patients with hemiplegia. While the incidence of RSD appears to range between 12–32%, Petchkrua et al. (2002) suggested that the incidence of RSD is over-estimated and the results from previous studies were obtained before patients routinely received early intensive inpatient rehabilitation. At admission to hospital and one week until discharge, patients admitted to an acute rehabilitation facility, were evaluated for shoulder pain, decreased passive range of motion of the shoulder, wrist/ hand pain, edema, and skin changes. If three of these five criteria were positive, patients underwent a triple-phase bone scan (TPBS). Bone scan findings consistent with CRPS type 1 were taken as confirming the diagnosis. Of 64 subjects, 13 underwent bone scans, with only one (1.56%) positive result. The authors noted it was possible that patients were discharged before they developed symptoms of RSD. Patients from a more recent study (Kondo et al. 2001) who received standard multidisciplinary rehabilitation had a much higher incidence of RSD (34%). Gokkaya et al. (2006) were the more recent investigators to suggest that there was a relationship between RSD and shoulder subluxation. Possible mechanisms suggested by the authors included overstretching of periarticular tissues and impingement on the nerve tissues and downward traction of the shoulder joint complex.

Conclusion

The incidence of RSD poststroke ranges from 12–34% and may be influenced by the timing as well as the type of assessment.

Diagnostic Tests of SHS

Several approaches to diagnose RSD have been used. Routine radiographs of the involved upper extremity may demonstrate a patchy, periarticular demineralization (Sudek's atrophy) as early as 3–6 months after the onset of clinical signs. The most sensitive diagnostic test is the technetium diphosphonate bone scan which demonstrates increased periarticular uptake (mostly at the shoulder and wrist) in the affected upper extremity. Bone scan abnormalities appear earlier than the X-ray changes. Tepperman et al. (1984) found 25% of hemiplegic patients demonstrated evidence of reflex sympathetic dystrophy in the involved upper extremity although only two-thirds went on to develop the clinical syndrome. Temporary resolution of symptoms with sympathetic blockade is considered diagnostic despite potential difficulties with the technique in terms of diagnostic validity. Thermography, in controlled studies, has failed to consistently diagnose reflex sympathetic dystrophy and is not considered a valid test. However, Kozin et al. (1981) suggested that clinical measurement such as grip strength, tenderness and ring size were more accurate diagnostic indicator of RSD. Iwate et al. (2002) have suggested that a ratio of the circumference of the middle finger (affected; unaffected) greater than 1.06 at four weeks post-stroke was predictive of RSD.

Conclusion

Shoulder hand syndrome is a painful clinical entity, which is not understood from a pathophysiological basis. The diagnosis is made clinically. Most cases appear to improve with time.

Treatment of Shoulder-Hand Syndrome

Prevention of shoulder problems and aggressive early treatment are recommended to prevent the development of a non-functional painful upper extremity. To prevent shoulder hand syndrome, prevent shoulder subluxation, maintain JROM of the extremity by active and passive exercises. Modalities such as contrast bath, interferential therapy, deep heating modalities, TENS are used for the treatment of RSD. Sometimes resting hand and wrist splint is also recommended. Medications such as analgesics, NSAIDs, high dose corticosteroids can be tried. In case it does not respond to medical treatment sympathetic block and finally sympathectomy can be tried.

Therapy consists of vigorous physiotherapy with a focus on range of motion exercises. A one to two week course of high dose corticosteroids and/or sympathetic blocks either in the form of stellate ganglion blocks or guanethedine local venous blocks may be tried in persistent disabling cases. Constraint-induced movement therapy and sensory discrimination training have also been proposed as possible treatments for SHS (Acerra et al. 2007). A surgical sympathectomy may be considered if stellate ganglion sympathetic blocks are consistently effective but symptoms recur. However, there is no evidence that surgical sympathectomy alter outcomes. There is no definitive therapeutic intervention for reflex sympathetic dystrophy, as reflected by the large number of suggested treatments. Shoulder hand syndrome, which presents for greater than 6 months without appropriate treatment, has a poor prognosis (Lieberman 1986).

The study by Braus et al. (1994) was the only RCT examining a treatment for shoulder-hand syndrome. Oral corticosteroids improved SHS for at least 4 weeks. Despite a limited number of trials, a review by Geurts et al. (2000) concluded that oral corticosteroids were the most effective treatment for SHS. While a single controlled trial found that calcitonin treatment effectively treated pain associated with SHS, it is not widely used clinically.

Conclusion

There is moderate (Level 1b) evidence that oral corticosteroids improve shoulder-hand syndrome for at least the first 4 weeks.

There is limited (level 2) evidence that calcitonin improves pain associated with SHS following stroke. Oral corticosteroids appear to improve shoulder-hand syndrome for at least the first 4 weeks.

Graded Motor Imagery

Motor imagery has been suggested as an alternative therapy to conventional medical management of SHS and involves activation of cortical networks without initially involving movement of the affected limb. A versoin of this strategy (mirror therapy) has been used successfully for patients suffering from phantom pain. There may be an association between CRPS and a neglect-like condition, such that patients may need to focus their attention to move the affected limb (Moseley et al. 2004). The mechanisms underlying motor imagery remain unclear, although it is known that both real and imagined movements activate similar cortical networks. Proposed mechanisms include reconciliation of motor output and sensory feedback, activation of mirror neurons and graded activation of cortical motor networks (Acerra et al. 2007). A single RCT evaluated the effectiveness of this treatment following stroke.

In the first phase of the treatment hand laterality recognition, avoidance of activation of the primary motor cortex was achieved by only initiating activation in the pre-motor cortices. In the second stage, patients were asked to imagine their own hand placed in the same position as a picture selected from 28 pictures chosen at random. In the final stage, pictures of the unaffected hand were placed into a cardboard mirror box. Patients were asked to adopt the posture in the picture (n=20) times with both hands, but to discontinue if they experienced pain.

Mosele, et al. (2004) reported that treatment with MIP was more effective than ongoing medical management. Patients experienced significant reductions in pain and swelling associated with treatment, which persisted for at least 6 weeks. The authors also noted that 6 weeks after completing the MIP program, approximately 50% of patients no longer fulfilled the diagnostic criteria for CRPS1.

Conclusion

There is moderate (level 1b) evidence that a modified imagery program can reduce pain associated with shoulder-hand syndrome. A motor imagery program appears to improve shoulder-hand syndrome.

SUMMARY

1. Shoulder subluxation occurs early following a stroke.
2. Hemiplegic shoulder pain is associated with shoulder subluxation and spasticity, but not with scapular rotation.
3. There appears to be an important role for the subscapularis muscle and to a lesser extent pectoralis major musculature, which develop greater tonic activity on the hemiparetic side with subsequent muscle limbalance about the shoulder.
4. The development of painful hemiplegic shoulder is associated with severe strokes and poorer functional outcome.
5. There is moderate (Level 1b) evidence that prolonged positioning does not negatively influence shoulder range of motion or pain.
6. There is limited (Level 2) evidence that shoulder slings prevent subluxation associated with hemiplegic shoulder pain, although there is also limited (Level 2) evidence that one device or method is better than another.
7. There is conflicting (Level 4) evidence that strapping the hemiplegic shoulder reduces the development of pain. There is moderate (Level 1b) evidence that strapping the hemiplegic shoulder does not improve range of motion or upper limb function.
8. There is moderate (Level 1b) evidence that the use of overhead pullies results in surprisingly high levels of hemiplegic shoulder pain and should be avoided.

9. There is moderate (Level 1b) evidence that a gentle range of motion program by a therapist results in less hemiplegic shoulder pain.
10. There is moderate (Level 1b) evidence that corticosteroid injections do not improve shoulder pain or range of motion in hemiplegic patients. There is limited (Level 2) evidence that oral non-steroidal anti-inflammatories can reduce pain during therapy sessions. There is limited (Level 2) evidence that botulinum toxin can reduce pain in the hemiplegic shoulder.
11. There is conflicting (Level 4) evidence that functional electrical stimulation reduces pain, improves function and reduces subluxation following stroke.
12. There is moderate (Level 1b) evidence that motor blocks of the subscapular muscle reduces spastic shoulder pain and improves passive range of motion of the hemiplegic shoulder.
13. There is conflicting (Level 4) evidence that motor blocks of the pectporalis major muscle reduces spastic shoulder pain or improves passive range of motion of the hemiplegic shoulder.
14. There is moderate (Level 1b) evidence that aromatherapy combined with acupressure can reduce pain associated with painful hemiplegic shoulder.
15. Shoulder hand syndrome is a poorly understood clinical entity. Most cases improve with time.
16. There is moderate (Level 1b) evidence that oral corticosteroids improve shoulder hand syndrome for at least the first 4 weeks.
17. There is moderate (Level 1b) evidence that modified imagery program can reduce pain associated with shoulder-hand syndrome. There is limited (Level 2) evidence that calcitonin improves pain associated with SHS following stroke.

BIBLIOGRAPHY

1. Acerra NE, Souvlis T, Moseley GL. Stroke, complex regional pain syndrome and phantom limb pain: can commonalities direct future management? J Rehabil Med. 2007;39:109-14.

2. Ada L, Foongchmcheay A. Efficacy of electrical stimulation in preventing reducing subluxation of the shoulder after stroke: a meta-analysis. Aust J Physiother 2002;48(4):257-67.
3. Ada L, Goddard E McCully, J, Stavrinos T, Bampton J. Thirty minutes of positioning reduces the development of shoulder external rotation contracture after stroke: A randomized controlled trial. Arch Phys Med Rehabil 2005;86:230-4.
4. Ada L, Foongchomcheay A, Canning C. Supportive devices for preventing and treating subluxation of the shoulder after stroke. Cochrane Database Syst Rev 2005;CD003863.
5. Ancliffe J. Strapping the shoulder in patients following a cerebrovascular accident (CVA): A pilot study. Australian Journal of Physiotherapy 1992;38:37-9.
6. Aras MD, Gokaya NK, Comert D, Kaya A, Cakci A. Shoulder pain in hemiplegia: results form a national rehabilitation hospital in Turkey. Am J Phys Med Rehabil 2004;83:713-9.
7. Arsenault AB, Silodean M, Duil E, Riley E. Clinical significance of the V-shaped space in the subluxed shoulder of hemiplegics. Stroke 1991;22:867-1.
8. Baker LL, Parker K. Neuromuscular electrical stimulation of the muscles surrounding the shoulder. Phys Ther 1986;66:1990-37.
9. Basmajian JV, Bazant FJ. Factors preventing downward dislocation of adducted shoulder joint: electromyographic and morphological study. J bone Joint Surg (Am) 1959;41:1182-6.
10. Bender L, Mckenna K. Hemiplegic shoulder pain: Defining the problem and its management. Disability and Rehabilitation 2001;23(16):698-705.
11. Bhakta BB, Cozens JA, Bamford JM, Chamberalin M. Use of botulinum toxin in stroke patients with severe upper limb spasticity. J Neurol Neurosurg Psychiatr 1996;6130-5.
12. Bloch R, Bayer N. Prognosis in stroke. Cl Orthop Related Res 1978; 131:10-14.
13. Bobath B. Adult hemiplegia: Evaluation and assessment (3rd ed). Heinemann, London, 1990.
14. Bohannon RW. Relationship between shoulder pain and selected variable in patients with hemiplegia. Clinical Rehabilitation 1988;2:111-7.
15. Bohannon RW, Andrews AW. Shoulder subluxation and pain in stroke patients. American J Occup Therapy 1990;44(6):507-9.
16. Bohannon RW, Larkin PA, Smith MB, Horton MG. Shoulder pain in hemiplegia: statistical relationship with five variables. Arch Phys Med Rehabil 1986;67:514-6.
17. Boyd EA. Clinical measures of shoulder subluxation: their reliability. Can J Public Health 1992;83 Suppl 2:524-8.

18. Braun RM, West Flower, Mooney V, Nickel RL, Roper B, Caldwell C. Surgical treatment of the painful shoulder contracture in the stroke patient. J Bone Joint Surg (Am) 1971;53:1307-12.
19. Braus DF, Krauss JK, strobel J. The shoulderhand syndrome after stroke: a clinical trial. Ann Neurol 1994;36(5):728-33.
20. Brooke MM, de Lateur BJ, Diana - Rigby GC, Questad KA. Shoulder subluxation in hemiplegia: effects of three different supports. Arch Phys Med Rehabil 1991;72:582-6.
21. Cailliet R. The shoulder in hemiplegia. Philadelphia, PA, FA. Davis Co., 1980.
22. Caldwell CB, Wilson DJ, Brown RM. Evaluation and treatment of the upper extremity in the hemiplegic stroke patient. Clin Orthop, 1969;63:69-93.
23. Carr EK, Kenney FD. Positioning of the stroke patient: a review of the literature. Int J Nurs. Stud, 1992;29(4):355-69.
24. Chaco J, Wolf E. Subluxation of the glenohumeral joint in hemiplegia. Am J Phys Med, 1971;50:139-43.
25. Chae J, Yu DT, Walker ME, et al, Intramuscular Electrical Stimulation for Hemiplegic Shoulder Pain: A 12- Month Follow - up of a Multiple - Canter, Randomized Clinical Trial. Am J Phys Med Rehabil, 2005; 84:832-42.
26. Chantraine A, Baribeault A, Uebelhart D, Gremion G. Shoulder pain and dysfunction in hemiplegia: effects of functional electrical stimulation. Arch Phys Med Rehabil 1999;80:328-31.
27. Church C, Price C, Pandyan AD, Huntley S, Curies R, Rodgers H. Randomized Controlled Trial to Evaluate the Effect of Surface Neuromuscular Electrical Stimulation to the Shoulder After Acute Stoke. Stroke 2006;37:2995-3001.
28. Codman EA. The Shoulder. Boston, Thomas Todd Co, 1934.
29. Cole TM, Tobis JS. Measurement of musculoskeletal function. In: Kotke FJ, Lehmann JF (eds). Krusen's Handbook of Physical Medicine and Rehabilitation. Philadelphia, Saunders, p. 25, 1990.
30. Crossens-Sills J, Schenkman M. Analysis of shoulder pain, range of motion, and subluxation in patients with hemiplegia. Phys. Ther, 1985;65:731.
31. Culham EG, Noce RR, Bagg SD. Shoulder complex position and glenohumeral subluxation in hemiplegia. Arch Phys Med Rehabil, 1995;76:856-64.
32. Davis SW, Pestrillo CR, Eischberg RD, Chu DS. Shoulder - hand syndrome in a hemiplegic population: a 5-year retrospective study. Arch Phys Med Rehab, 1977;58:353-5.
33. Dean CM,Mackey FH, Katrak P. Examination of shoulder positioning after stroke: A randomized controlled pilot trial. Australian Journal of Physiotherapy, 2000;46:35-40.

34. De Jong LD, Nieuwboer A, Aufdemakampe G. Contracture preventive positioning of he hemiplegic arm in subacute stroke patients: a pilot randomized controlled trial. Clin Rehabil. 2006; 20:656-67.
35. Dekker JH, Wagenaar RC, Landhorst GJ, de Jong BA. The painful hemiplegic shoulder: effects of intraarticular triamcinolone acetonide. Am J Phys Med Rehabil, 1997;76:43-8.
36. Eto F, Yoshikawa M, Ueda S, Hirai S. Post-hemiplegic shoulder-hand syndrome with special reference to related cerebral localization. J Am Ger Soc, 1980;2813-7.
37. Faghi PD. The effects of neuromuscular stimulation induced muscle contraction versus elevation on hand edema in CVA patients. J Hand Ther, 1997;10:29-34.
38. Feghri PD, Rodgers MM, Glaser RM, Bors JG, Ho C, Akuthota P. The effects of functional electrical stimulation on shoulder subluxation, arm function recovery, and shoulder pain in hemiplegic stroke patients. Arch Phys Med Rehabil, 1994;75:73-9.
39. Fizgeraild -Finch OP, Gibson II: Subluxation of shoulder in hemiplegia. Age Ageing, 1975;4(1):16-8.
40. Fugl-Meyer AR, Jaasko L, Leyman I, Oisson S, Steglind S. Post-stroke hemiplegic patient: I Method for evaluation of physical performance. Scand J Rehab Med, 1975;7(1):13-31.
41. Gamble GE, Barberan E, Laasch HU, Bowsher D, Tyrell PJ, Jones AK, poststroke shoulder pain: a prospective study of the association and risk factors in 152 patients form a consecutive cohort of 205 patients presenting with stroke. Eur J Pain, 2002;6: 467-74.
42. Geurts A, Visschers B, Van Limbeek J, Ribbers G. Systematic review of aetiology and treatment of poststroke hand edema and shoulder-hand syndrome. Scan J Rehab Med, 2000;32:4-10.
43. Gilmore, PE, Spaulding SJ, Vandervoort AA. Hemiplegic shoulder pain: Implications for occupational therapy treatment. Can J Occup Ther, 2004;71(1)36-46.
44. Gokkaya Nk, Aras M, Yesiltepe E, et al. Reflex sympathetic dystrophy in hemiplegia. Int J Rehabil Res, 2006;29:275-9.
45. Griffin A, Berhnhardt J. Strapping the hemiplegic shoulder prevents development of pain during rehabilitation: a randomized controlled trail. Clin Rehabil, 2006;20(A):287-95.
46. Gresham GE, Duncan PW, Staston WB, et al. Post-Stroke Rehabilitation Guideline. Post-stroke Rehabilitation. Clinical Practice Guideline No. 16 CAHCRP Publication No. 95-0662), Rockville, MD: US. Department of Health and Human Services, Public Health service, agency for Health Care Policy and Research, May 1995.

47. Griffin A, Bernhardt J. Strapping the hemiplegic shoulder prevents development of pain during rehabilitation: a randomized controlled trial. Clin Rehabil, 2006;(4):287-95.
48. Gustafsson L, McKenna K. A programme of static positional stretches does not reduce hemiplegic shoulder pain or maintain shoulder range of motion-a randomized controlled trial. Clin Rehabil, 2006;20(4):277-86.
49. Hakuno A, Sashika H, Ohkawa T, Itoh R. Arthrographic findings in hemiplegic shoulders. Arch Phys Med Rehab, 1984;65:706-11.
50. Hamamci N, Dursun E, Ural C, Cakci A. Calcitonin treatment in reflex sympathetic dystrophy: a preliminary study. Br J Clin Pract, 1996;50(7):373-5.
51. Hanger HC, Whitewood P, Brown G, Ball MC, Harper J, Cox R, Sainsbury R. A. randomized controlled trial of strapping to prevent post-stroke shoulder pain. Clin Rehabil 2000;14:370-80.
52. Hecht JS. Subscapular nerve block I the painful hemiplegic shoulder. Arch Phsy Med Rehabil 1992;73:1036-9.
53. Hecht JS. The role of spasticity in hemiplegic shoulder pain and what to do about it. 57th Annual Assembly of American Academy of Physical Medicine and Rehabilitation, Oriando, Florida, November 17, 1995,pp.248-55.
54. Hollinshead WH, Jenkins DB. Functional anatomy of the limbs. Philadelphia Saunders, 1981.p.105.
55. Hurd MM, Farrel KH, Waylonis GW. Shoulder sling for hemiplegia: friend or foe? Arch Phys Med Rehabil 1974;5:5519-22.
56. Ikai T, Tei K, Oshida K, Miyano S, Yonemoto K. Evaluation and treatment of shoulder subluxation in hemiplegia: relationship between subluxation and pain. Am J Phys Med Rehabil, 1998;77(5): 421-6.
57. Inaba MK, Piorkowski M. Ultrasound in treatment of painful shoulder in patients with hemiplegia. J Phys Ther, 1972;52:737-41.
58. Iwata M, Kondo I, Sato Y, Satoh K, soma M, Br-OrO. Prediction of reflex sympathetic dystrophy in hemiplegia by evaluation of hand edema. Arch Phys Med Rehabil, 2002;83(10):1428-31.
59. Janig W, Baron R. Complex regional pain syndrome is a disease of the central nervous system. Clin Auton Res 2002;12:150-64.
60. Johnstone M. The stroke patient: Principles of rehabilitation. Churchill Livingstone, Edinburgh, 1982.
61. Joynt RL. The source of shoulder pain in hemiplegia. Arch Phys Med Rehabil, 1992;73:409-13.
62. Kaplan M. Hemiplegic shoulder pain early prevention and rehabilitation. West J Med, 1995.
63. Kaplan PE, Meredith J, Taft G, Betts HB. Stroke and brachial plexus injury: A difficult problem. Arch Phys Med Rehab, 1977;38:415-8.

64. Kingery WS, Date ES, Bobobo CR. The absence of brachial plexus injury in stroke. AM Phys Med Rehab, 1993;72:127-75.
65. Kobayashi H, Onishi H, Ihashi K, Yagi R, Handa Y. Reduction in subluxation and improved muscle function of the hemiplegic shoulder joint after therapeutic electrical stimulation. J Electromyogr kinesiol, 1999;9:327-36.
66. Kondo I, Hosokawa K, Soma M, Iwata M, Maltais D. Protocol to prevent shoulder - hand syndrome after stroke. Arch Phys Med Rehabil, 2001;82(11):1619-23.
67. Kong KH, Neo JJ, Chua KS. A randomized controlled study of botulinum toxin A in the treatment of hemiplegic shoulder pain associated with spasticity. Clin Rehabil, 2007;21:28-35.
68. Kozin F, McCarty D, Sims J. Genant H. Reflex sympathetic dystrophy: I. Clinical and histological studies: evidence for bilaterality, response to corticosteroids and articular involvement. Am J Med 1976;60:332-8 (b).
69. Kozin F, Genant HK, Bekerman C, McCarty DJ. Reflex sympathetic dystrophy syndrome: II. Roentenographic and scintigraphic evidence of bilaterality and of periarticular accentuation. Am J Med 1976;60:332-8(b).
70. Kozin F, Ryan LM, Carrera GF, Soin JS, Wortman RL. Reflex sympathetic dystrophy syndrome (RSDS): III Scintigraphic studies, further evidence for the therapeutic efficacy of systemic corticosteroids, and proposed diagnostic criteria. Am J Med, 1981; 70:23-30.
71. Kozin F. Two unique shoulder disorders: Adhesive capsulitis and reflex sympathetic dystrophy syndrome. Postgrad Med, 1983; 73:207-16.
72. Kumar R, Metter EJ, Mehta AJ, Chew T. Shoulder pain in hemiplegia. The role of exercise. Am J Phys Med Rehabil, 1990;69(4): 205-8.
73. Lieberman JS. Hemiplegia: Rehabilitation of the upper extremity. In: Kaplan PE, Cerullo LJ (Eds.): Stroke rehabilitation. Stoneman, MA, Butter worth Publishers, 1986;95-115.
74. Lindgren I, Jonsson AC, Norrving B, et al, Shoulder pain after stroke: a prospective population - based study. Stroke. 2007;38:343-48.
75. Linn SL, Granat MH, Lees KR. Prevention of shoulder subluxation after stroke with electrical stimulation. Stroke 1999;30:963-8.
76. Lo SF, Chen SY, Lin HC, Jim YF Meng, NH Kao MJ. Arthrographic and clinical findings in patients with hemiplegic shoulder pian. Arch Phys Med Rehabil 2003;84:1786-91.
77. Lynch D, Feraro M, Krol J, Trudell CM, Christos P, Volpe BT. Continuous passive motion improves shoulder joint integrity following stroke. Clin Rehabil 2005;19:594-9.

78. Marco E, Duarte E, Vila J, et al. Is botulinum toxin type A effective in the treatment of spastic shoulder pain in patients after stroke? A double-blind randomized clinical trial. J Rehabil Med. 2007;39: 440-47.
79. Moodie NB, Brishbin J, Morgan AM. Subluxation of the gleno-humeral joint in hemiplegia: Evaluation of supportive devices. Physiotherapy Canada 1986;38:151-7.
80. Morin L, Bravo G. Strapping the hemiplegic shoulder: A radio-graphic evaluation of its efficacy to reduce subluxation. Physiotherapy Canada 1997;49:103-8.
81. Moseley GL. Graded motor imagery is effective for long-standing complex regional pain syndrome: a randomized controlled trial. Pain, 2004;108:192-8.
82. Moskowitz E. Complications in rehabilitation of hemiplegic patients. Med Clin North Am, 1969;53:541-99(a).
83. Moskowitz E, Goodman CR, Smith E, Bathazar E, Mellins HZ. Hemiplegic shoulder. NY State J Med 1969;69:548-50(b).
84. Najenson T, Yacubovich E, Pikelini S. Rotator cuff injury in hemiplegic patients. Scand J Rehab Med, 1971;3:131-7.
85. Nepomuceno CS, Miller JM III. Shoulder arthrography in hemiplegic patients. Arch Phys Med Rehab Med Rehab, 1974;55: 49-51.
86. Paci M, Nannetti L, Rinaldi LA. Glenohumeral subluxation in hemi-plegia: an overview. J Rehabil Res Dev 2005;42(4)557-68.
87. Partridge CJ, Edwards SM, Mee R, Van Langenberghe HV. Hemiplegic shoulder pain: a study of two methods of physio-therapy treatment. Clinical Rehabilitation 1990;4:43-9.
88. Patterson JR, Zabransky R, Grabois M, Ferro P. Evaluation of the effectiveness of sling orthoses for the correction of glenohumeral subluxation in the hemiplegic. Archives Phys Med Rehabil, 1984; 65:35.
89. Pperrigot M, Bussel B, Peirrot Deseilligny E, Held JP. L'epaule de I' hemiplegique. Am Med Phys, 1975;18:175-87.
90. Poduri KR. Shoudler pain in stroke patients and its effects on rehabilitation. J Stroke Cerebrovasc Dis, 1993;3261-6.
91. Post MW, Visser-Meily JM, Boomkamp-Koppen HG, Prevo AJ. Assessment of oedema in stroke patients: comparison of visual inspection by therapists and volumetric assessment. Disabil Rehabil, 2002;25:1265-70.
92. Poulin De Courval L, Barsauskas A, Berenbaum B, Dehaut Flower, Dussault R, Fontaine FS, Labrecque R, Leclerc C, Girous F. Painful shoulder in the hemiplegic and unilateral neglect. Arch Phys Med Rehabil, 1990; 71(9):673-6.

93. Prevost R, Arsenault AB, Dutil E, Drouin G. Rotation of the scapular and shoulder subluxation in hemiplegia. Arch Phys Med Rehab, 1987;68:786-90.
94. Price CL, Pandyan AD. Electrical stimulation for preventing and treating post-stroke shoulder pain: a systematic Cochrane review. Clin Rehabil, 2001;15:5-19.
95. Rizk TE, Christopher RP, Pinals RS, Salazar JE, Higgins C. Arthrographic studies in painful hemiplegic shoulders. Arch Phys Med Rehab, 1984; 65:254-5.
96. Rommel O, Malin JP, Zenz M, Janig W. Quantitative sensory testing, neurophysiological and psychological examination in patients with complex regional pain syndrome and hemisensory deficits. Pain 2001;93:279-93.
97. Roper TA, Redford S, Tallis RC. Intermittent compression for the treatment of the oedematous hand in hemiplegic stroke: a randomized controlled trial. Age Ageing, 1999;29:9-13.
98. Roy CW, Sands M, Hill L, Harrison, Marshall S. The effect of shoulder pain on outcome of acute hemiplegia. Clin Rehabil, 1995; 9:21-7.
99. Roy CW, Sands MR, Hill LD. Shoulder pain in acutely admitted hemiplegics. Clinical Rehabilitation, 1996;18:359-501.
100. Renzenbrink GJ, Ijzerman MJ. Percutaneous neuromuscular electrical stimulation (P-NMES) for treating shoulder pain in chronic hemiplegia. Effects on shoulder pain and quality of life. Clin Rehabil, 2004;18:359-65.
101. Savage R, Robertson L. Relationship between adult hemiplegic shoulder pain and depression. Physiotherapy Can 1982; 34:86-90.
102. Shahani BT, Kelly EB, Glasser S. Hemiplegic shoulder subluxation. Arch Phys Med Rehab, 1981;62:519.
103. Shai G, Ring H, Costeff H, Solzi P. Glenohumeral misalignment in hemiplegic shoulder. Scan J Rehab Med, 1984;16:133-6.
104. Shin BC, Lee MS. Effects of aromatherapy acupressure on hemiplegic shoulder pain and motor power in stroke patients: a pilot study. J Altern Complement Med. 2007;13:247-51.
105. Sneis IA, Beckerman H, Twisk JW, Dekker JH, Peter DK, Koppe PA, Lankhorst GJ, Bouter LM. Effect of triamcinolone acetonide injections of hemiplegic shoulder pain: A randomized clinical trial. Stroke, 2000;31:296-2401.
106. Steinbrocker D. Shoulder hand syndrome: present perspective. Arch Phys Med Rehab, 1969;49:388-95.
107. Tahmoush AJ. Causalgia: redefinition as a clinical pain syndrome. Pain, 1981;10:187.
108. Teppermna PS, Greyson ND, Hilbert L, et al. Reflex sympathetic dystrophy in hemiplegia. Arch Phys Med Rehab, 1984;65(8):442-7.

109. Tyson SF and Chissim C. The immediate effect of handling technique on range of movement in the hemiplegic shoulder. Clinical Rehabilitation, 2002;16:137-40.
110. Van Ouwenwaller C, Laplace PM, Chantraine A. Painful shoulder in hemiplegia. Arch Phys Med Rehabil, 1986;67:23-6.
111. Walsh K. Management of shoulder pain in patients with stroke. Postgrad Med J, 2001;77:645-9.
112. Wang RY, Chan RC, Tsai MW. Functional electrical stimulation on chronic and acute hemiplegic shoulder subluxation. Am J Phys Med Rehabil, 2000;79:385-90.
113. Wanklyn P, Forester A, Young J. Hemiplegics shoulder pain (HSP): natural history and investigation of associated features. Disability and Rehabilitation 1996;18:497-501.
114. Williams R, Taffs L, Minuk T. Evaluation of two support methods for the subluxated shoulder of hemiplegic patients. Phys Ther 1988;68:1209-14.
115. Yeinik Ap, Colle FM, Bonan IV, Vicaut E. Treatment of shoulder pain in spastic hemiplegia by reducing spasticity of the subscapular muscle: A randomized, double-blind, placebo-controlled study of botulinum toxin. AJ Neurol Neurosurg Psychiatry, 2006.
116. Yu DT, Chae J, Walker ME, Fang ZP. Percutaneous intramuscular neuromuscular electric stimulation for the treatment of shoulder subluxation and pain in patients with chronic hemiplegia: a pilot study. Arch Phsy Med Rehabil 2001;82:20-5.
117. Yu DT, Chae J, Walker ME, Hart RL, Petroski GF. Comparing stimulation-induced pain during percutaneous (intramuscular and transcutaneous neuromuscular electric stimulation for treatment shoulder subluxation in hemiplegia. Arch Phys Med Rehabil 2001; 82:756-60.
118. Zorowitz RD, Idank D, Lkai T, Hughes MB, Johnston MV. Shoulder subluxation after stroke: A comparison of four supports. Arch Phys Med Rehabil, 1995;76:763-71.
119. Zorowitz RD, Hughes MB, Idank D, Ikai T, Johston V. Shoulder pain and subluxation after stroke: Correlation or coincidence? American Journal of Occupational Therapy 1996;50:194-201.

Chapter

9

Throwing Athletic Injury

INTRODUCTION

Affections of shoulder girdle have been the ruin of many athletes, whose major forte was throwing sports such as javelin, discus, short put, baseball, volleyball, cricket and tennis.

Nicholas and Grossman analyzed 63 sports and developed a classification of body movement. Throwing was found to be the most commonly required movement in sports. Activities involving repetitive use of the arm above the horizontal level may result in several injuries in and around shoulder. Many a times these injuries seem to be resistant to the common treatment techniques. Here it becomes very important to know the cause and explore into more effective measures.

Rotator cuff tendonitis or strains are the most common injuries affecting an overhand athlete. This may be due to either tensile loading or sudden injury. Treatment often focuses at improving joint motion, muscle force generating capacity and pain reduction.

The technique of throwing involves high forces that are applied to the shoulder within a short span of time. Throughout the movement, the shoulder muscles should work in asynchrony with proximal, i.e, scapular muscles. Rotator cuff muscles form an important part of shoulder to function as stabilizers and rotators. The proper biomechanical synchrony of the glenohumeral joint and the scapulothoracic joint during movement is crucial, which is disturbed by certain functional errors like improper techniques or muscle strength. This may go to such extent that they may impinge the important structures of shoulder. In an overhand athlete functional causes include lateral scapular slide and posterior capsule tightness and rotator cuff weakness. These factors, if present, will impinge on the already injured or inflamed, swollen rotator cuff leading to microtrauma and delayed repair. Thus, the treatment of the tendons cannot be effective till these interruptions are under control. Functional factors of impingement stated above can effectively be managed by physiotherapy.

A proper scapular position is a vital factor in the treatment of rotator cuff injuries. Scapular stabilization exercises, strengthening of scapular stabilizing muscles and regaining the scapulohumeral rhythm forms a basic tool to deal with such case. Flexibility also forms a main concern.

BIOMECHANICS AND PATHOKINESIOLOGY OF PITCHING

Throwing action is one of the most common movements of sports. The pattern is almost same in all types of sports. It is generally classified into 4 stages:

The preparation for a throw in the shoulder starts with *winding up*. Shoulder goes into abduction, extension and external rotation. The position of fingers on the ball is finalized. The EMG activity of the shoulder girdle and upper extremities is low during windup. The importance of the windup is that it sets up the body and arm position for the violent act of throwing to follow.

This phase is followed by cocking. It involves the throwing arm moving into full external rotation in about 90° of abduction. It is characterized by strong contraction of the external rotators of the shoulder joint in order to store elastic energy in the recoil system. This activity of the posterior deltoid, supra and infraspinatus and teres minor muscles continue until the explosive medial rotation of the humerus signifies the onset of the acceleration phase. The upper trapezius rotates the scapula upwards to place the glenoid in a stable position for abducting humeral head. The deltoid and the supra- spinatus concomitantly abduct the humeral head. During late cocking, rapid forward rotating motion of the shoulder is noted. This phase place the glenohumeral capsule (and cuff) in maximum lateral rotation and horizontal extension at 90° of abduction (90° abduction in 30° horizontal extension and 90° external rotation). In this position, the capsule and the cuff of the joint are under stress from sources. Firstly, the torsion effect on the rotation wrings the capsule posteriorly placing stress on the upper rotator cuff tendons. Secondly, the strong contraction of the posterior fibers of the deltoid lever the head of the humerus anteriorly hard against the anterior labrum and cuff. The short external rotators of the cuff (teres minor and infraspinatus) must work hard to prevent the humeral head from migrating forward under the force of the deltoid. In this phase inertia and gravity act on the arm in horizontal abduction, external rotation and adduction, however the arm does not move in the direction of these forces. Cocking takes place approximately in 1.5 seconds. Large torque is generated in the shoulder to overcome the above forces. Static and dynamic restraints combine to stabilize the joint against these forces. In this position, the primary anterior stabilizer of the glenohumeral joint is the anterior inferior glenohumeral ligament. The scapulothoracic muscles protract and rotate the scapula upward to produce a stable platform for the humeral head, thus enhancing maximal humeral external rotation. The muscles activity during the cocking phase involves deltoid, supraspinatus, infraspinatus and teres minor and then subscapularis (Jobe et al. 1983). During cocking, posterior excursion of the throwing arm to approximately 30° of extension in the horizontal plane, combined with shoulder girdle rotation is necessary so that accelerating force may be applied to the ball more efficiently. Extension in horizontal plane results by the posterior deltoid action on middle trapezius and rhomboids construction adducting the scapula. The serratus anterior stabilizes the scapula against the chest wall.

In the latter moments of the cocking position, the humerus is brought forward from 30° extension to a neutral position in the horizontal plane. At this point, the scapula abducts to neutral from its adducted position to allow for forward horizontal movement of the humerus.

Next to this, is the acceleration phase that comprises 2% of the pitching sequence. The acceleration phase begins with maximal shoulder external rotation (40-60° at ball release) and terminates with ball release. It consists of explosive medial rotation and forward translation of the humerus. This phase must be efficient for a maximum transfer of momentum. The angular velocities achieved during expert throwing are extremely high, in the order of 6000–7000° per second. At late cocking, there is a lateral rotation torque of around 17600 joules, upon acceleration the torque reverses to an internal rotatory force of around 18900 Joules. Peak angular velocity is 5 m/s before ball release. Following the release of the object, the external rotators decelerate the arm by producing yet another torque reversal of similar magnitude. These 3 cycles of loading/unloading occur within 1/10 of a second. The acceleration phase is powerful but short lived lasting around 50 ms in expert throwers. The latissimus dorsi and pectoralis major produce the medial rotation with little activity of the subscapularis. The scapula is stabilized by serratus anterior, meanwhile infraspinatus, teres minor and supraspinatus are activated to stabilize the humeral head in the glenoid. These actions should assist in minimizing the subacromial impingement that can occur during acceleration. The middle trapezius and the rhomboids eccentrically contract to hold the scapula rotated up and to move the scapula lateral in a controlled manner. The upper trapezius and levator scapulae elevate the scapula along with a slightly upward rotatory effect.

Acceleration phase is followed by follow through. This phase comprises approximately 18% of the pitching sequence, here the shoulder girdle moves into horizontal flexion and internal rotation. Eccentric contraction of posterior deltoid and rotator cuff occur. In addition, eccentric contraction of middle trapezius, rhomboids, pectoralis major and latissimus dorsi occurs. Follow through occurs in approximately 350 m. The internal rotation of shoulder is approximately 30°. Later part of follow through is passive and due to the momentum.

In summary, the throwing motion requires the rapid transmission of large amounts of kinetic energy through the upper extremities. The resultant kinetic energy in the throwing arm has been estimated to 27,000 inch pounds, which is four times the energy in the leg during a soccer kick.

The performance of overhead sports activities like racket sports, javelin, volleyball, all have similar patterns. The excursion of the shoulder during a pitch is similar for all pitchers. Although details of mechanics of the entire throwing motion may vary, a thorough analysis reveals comparable patterns of movement in the glenohumeral, scapulothoracic and trunk complex. Recognition of the relationship of the moving segments to each other, i.e. humerus, scapula and trunk relation is essential.

Elevation of the arm is accomplished through glenohumeral and scapulothoracic interaction called "scapulohumeral rhythm". It requires both glenohumeral and scapulothoracic motion, which moves through 2:1 ratio of glenohumeral motion and scapular rotation. Malrotation or displacement of scapula is one of the most important factors to give rise to subacromial impingment. For every 10° of humeral elevation, there are 5° of clavicular elevation.

Intricate muscular force couples combine for stability and movements in glenohumeral joint, the forces contributing to scapular positioning are, force supporting weight of the extremity, the forces resisting scapular protraction and forces positioning the head of humerus into glenoid fossa. The force couples supporting the weight of extremity consists of upper fibers of trapezius, the levator scapule, the upper digitations of the serratus anterior, the rhomboids. The last 2 force couples combine their muscles and various lines of force to provide a wide variety of possible scapular positions. Of primary importance are the force couples that rotate the glenoid fossa upward. The upper and lower sections of trapezius and lower digits of serratus anterior are responsible for upward rotation. Stability in rotation is provided by rhomboids and trapezius along with pectoralis minor. Less scapular protraction is evident during abduction than flexion.

The vascularity of the rotator cuff has been a controversial subject for numerous years. Lindblom proposed that the rotator cuff is hypovascular or avascular near the suprapinatus attachment of the greater tuberosity. Codman referred to this vascular area as the "critical zone" where many lesions occur. Several others have reported under-vascularity in this zone. Moseley and Goldies, using microradiography and histology to study the vascular supply of the cuff, concluded that this area is not less vascular than the remainder of the cuff, but rather than this area represents the anastomoses between the osseous and tendinous vessels. Recent studies utilizing laser Doppler technique have revealed substantial blood flow in the critical area. Some authors have proposed compromise of supraspinatus blood flow based on arm movements. Rethbun and Macnab noted when the arm is adducted; it puts the tendon under tension and in effect causes a "wringing out" of the vessels. Sigholm et al reported a significant increase (by five folds) in subacromial pressure when the arm is elevated from 0° to 45°. If sustained, these pressures are sufficiently high to substantially reduce the tendon microcirculation.

There are numerous types of pathologies and injuries observed at the rotator cuff musculotendinous junction. Subacromial impingement appears to be one of the most common pathologies discussed. Impingement is defined as the "encroachment" of the rotator cuff (usually the supraspinatus) on the acromion, coracoacrominal ligament, coracoid process, and/or acromioclavicular joint as the shoulder is moved, particularly elevation and internal rotation. In 1972, Neer popularized the term "impingement," but the condition was recognized by many other clinicians such as Codman in 1972 and Armstrong, McLauglin, and Smith-Petersen at al in the 1940s. Nee at al. has described impingement as a progressive pattern involving a distinct three-stage process. In stage one; the lesions are described as a condition of cuff inflammation, edema, and hemorrhage, reversible with conservative treatment. In stage two, the lesion involves fibrosis and cuff tendinitis and may be treated conservatively. Stage three lesions involve bony changes (spurs) and cuff failure, necessitating surgical intervention.

Flatow et al. studies the contact of the rotator cuff on the undersurface of the acromion. The investigators used stereo-photogrammetry to determine contact areas while applying force along the rotator cuff and proximity was located at the anterolateral edge of the acromion at 0° elevation and shifted medially to the anteromedial adge with increasing arm elevation. In all cases (nine) and all test positions, contact involved only the anterior portion of the acromion. On the humeral side, contact was located at the proximal biceps region and supraspinatus tendon at 0° of elevation and shifted distally along these tendons with increasing arm, the authors noted contact was focused at the supraspinatus insertion. Furthermore, contact and proximity were consistently more pronounced in shoulder with a type III acromion or diminished external rotation. Thus in the normal shoulder, the rotator cuff particularly the supraspinatus and biceps, contact the acromion with arm elevation. The accumulative stresses over time in one region such as on the supraspinatus tendon may lead to failure.

Numerous factors may contribute to subacromial impingement. These factors have been classified as either structural or functional. Often these two factors are referred to as primary or secondary. In primary or structural impingement there is a structure that is responsible for the encroachment. The acromion is a commonly discussed site of impingement. If the acromion fails to ossify or unite, a condition referred to as os acromiale occurs. This results in a downward hanging acromion. Biglini at al have identified three types of acromion: type I (flat), type II (curved), and type III (hooked). Other structural factors such as degeneration or spurring of the acromioclavicular joint or the anterolateral acromion may cause impingement. Bursal inflammation or thickening or rotator cuff abnormalities may contribute as well.

Functional or secondary impingement occurs as a result of an underlying condition that causes the encroachment. There are three common mechanisms of functional impingement. Patients with subacromial impingement appear to exhibit a characteristic loss of motion pattern, described by Wilk and Andrews as a "reverse capsular pattern". Internal rotation is restricted the most and elevation second, with slight loss of external rotation. In this loss of motion patterns, usually the porterior capsule appears tight. Normal posterior capsular laxity allows the humeral head to stay centralized within the glenoid. Posterior capsular tightness results in an antero-superior migration of the humeral head and lateral slide of scapula causing encroachment of the humerus on the coraco-acromial ligament and/or acromion. Thus this impingement is secondary to capsular tightness; the treatment must be directed at normalizing the capsular flexibility.

In contrast, capsular hypermobility can also cause secondary impingement. If the capsule excessively lax and/or the dynamic stabilizers are inadequate, the humeral head will displace excessively, which may cause secondary impingement.

Hence, the successful treatment of subacromial impingement is based on a careful examination that identifies the causes of the pathology. Repetitive microtraumas are more of the causative factor for impingement than are macrotraumatic forces. Neer viewed impingement as a progressive degenerative process that often leads to failure of the rotator cuff.

Another example of impingement is acute traumatic impingement, which occurs secondary to a fall or diving for a ball in sports. The arm is usually abducted, extended, and internally rotated so that the force of the fall jams the humerus into the acromion and causes acute inflammation of the rotator cuff, bursae, and surrounding tissues. This type of injury responds well to non-operative treatment. In the older patient a thorough examination is necessary to exclude the possibility of a rotator cuff tear or avulsion of the cuff due to the forceful abduction.

Condition such as compressive cuff disease, tensile cuff failure, and/or posterior impingement may also develop secondary to glenohumeral joint instability.

The rotator cuff tendon or tendons may exhibit frank failure. There are many terms used to describe cuff tendon failure. Almost always the cuff fails near its periphery, near the attachment of the cuff to the tuberosity.

CLASSIFICATION OF INJURY

Cuff failure is described as partial or full-thickness tears. A full thickness tear extends all the way through from the articular surface to the bursal surface of the rotator cuff. Conversely, a partial-thickness tear involves only the superficial surface, mid-surface or deep surface. Acute tears occurring due to trauma account for approximately 3% to 8% of all rotator cuff tears. Chronic tears are those that have existed for a long time and are often insidious in onset and degenerative in nature. In addition, tears are characterized according to state of detachment from the humerus (retracted, atrophic or absent). Tears are also classified according to size of tears-small - less than 1 cm, medium - 1 to 3 cm, large - 3 to 5 cm and massive-greater than 5 cm.

Rotator cuff injury is one of the most common injuries at all activity levels in tennis players. However, recent investigations have pointed towards an alteration of the normal concept of this tendinitis. Although the classical symptoms and signs of crepitus and point tender pain over the anterior and lateral aspects of the shoulder upon overhead motion, which are relieved with the arm at the side, are usually present in most cases, there are probably two separate etiologies for these symptoms and signs.

In the athlete under 35 years of age, most of these symptoms are due to subclinical or mildly overt instabilities of the glenohumeral joint due to anterior inferior or anterior capsular and labral deficiencies. There rotator cuff injuries have been termed "secondary tensile overload injuries", because they occur as a result of deficits in muscular strength and balance and over-muscular inflexibility, which predispose to the capsular and labral deficiencies. Treatment in this group starts off with evaluation of flexibility and strength deficits that may be present, proceed with anterior, superior or multidirectional instability evaluation, and include tests for competence of all rotator cuff muscles. Conservative treatment that consists of decreased activity, range of motion exercises, which start at the scapula and work out to shoulder should be instituted first. In addition to the clinical symptom complex that has been described, treatment should be based on the complete analysis of all of the identified deficiencies.

Treatment of the symptomatic tendinitis may be limited by the anatomic instability, so if conservative treatment is not successful in progressing the athlete by 6 to 8 weeks, further evaluation by computed tomography (CT) arthrogram or magnetic resonance imaging (MRI) should be considered, to evaluate possible surgical cases. In these cases, the superior surface of the rotator cuff and subacromial space is usually not involved. The pathological problem will be found in the glenohumeral joint and on the undersurface of the rotator cuff.

In the older tennis athlete, the signs and symptoms are more commonly based on actual rotator cuff impingement and degeneration. In these patients the tendinits has been described as "primary compressive" because it is caused by damage directly to the cuff. A high percentage will show plain X-ray changes in the acromioclavicular (AC) joint, subacromial area, or greater tuberosity consistent with chronic wear. Tests for instability will usually be normal, but a pattern of strength imbalances similar to younger athletes may be present. Conservative treatment may be instituted, especially if there are a few indications of muscle tears. However, more complete diagnosis of the anatomic problem by arthrogram, CT arthrogram, or MRI should be considered early in the treatment process, so that accurate information about diagnosis, prognosis, treatment options, and return to play can be given.

Numerous factors contribute to cuff failure. Most full-thickness cuff tears appear to occur in tendons that have been weakened by some combination of age, repeated microtraumas, steroid injections, subacromial impingement, hypovascularity of the tendon, attrition, trauma and previous partial tearing.

The athletes most prone to acute supraspinatus tendinitis are swimmers, pitchers, weight lifters and throwers. At least 80% of swimmers have suffered from tendinitis of the supraspinatus at some time during their careers.

Asking a young athlete to throw repetitively or to go through motion while preparing for such athletic activity will easily produce rotator cuff tendinitis due to fatigue and muscle imbalance.

If the humeral head is not well contained in the shoulder socket by the internal and external rotators, or if the humeral head is not pulled back properly during throwing activity, the supraspinatus and biceps must compensate, which leads to fraying or breakdown of the supraspinatus at the greater tuberosity insertion. This usually produces a partial thickness internal rotator cuff tear. As the subluxation continues, that is, as the capsule gets looser over time, the humeral head tends to progressively migrate toward the acromion, leading to further erosion on the outside of the cuff. This will compress the bursa between acromion and cuff, leading to fibrosis initially and then breakdown ultimately.

Spurs and subacromial tissue thickening or remodeling into the type III acromial form may develop to stop concurrent subluxation or to act as a tissue space to centre the humeral head while the arm is down at the side. These compensatory mechanisms lead to progressive wear of the supraspinatus with overhead activity. Increased wobble of the glenohumeral joint due to wearing and stretching of the superior capsule and superior suspension mechanism stretching of the capsular of the underlying capsule causes synovitis of the posterior capsule, which leads to central stiffness and peripheral overuse of the scapulothoracic joint, all lead to further impingement. The actual pathology that occurs in the impingement area is a combination of inflammation, fibrosis and erosion. The bursa may be primarily inflamed. More commonly the cuff may be jammed up into the acromial surface either due to a fall or due to subluxation of the glenohumeral joint. A bony spur may develop in these locations; under the acromion at the origin of the coracoacromial ligament, from the coracoid at the insertion of the acromial origin of the deltoid tendon, or on either side of an arthritic AC joint, causing supraspinatus penetration. Spurs also develop at the rotator cuff insertion into the greater tuberosity due to microtrauma.

The serosal walls of the bursa, which attach to the coraco-acromial ligament have fine cross striations in youth but these usually degenerate in the early teenage years. Serosal walls may get inflamed showing mono and polymorphonucleocyte invasions in early athletic overuse and then thicken as cross-striation between the bursal walls, coalescence of the walls or erosion occurs. With repetitive use, the central subacromial bursa tends to wear out with peripheral thickening of wall and eventual separation of the subacromial space from the subdeltoid space. Coalescence of the wall may pull the rotator cuff up toward the acromion, increasing impingement.

Encroachement of bony spurs into the supraspinatus outlet wears into the rotator cuff, roughening its surface so that it no longer glides smoothly under the acromion. Such spurs commonly occur under the inferoanterior acromion, infero-posterior clavicle or the AC joint itself.

Histologic changes within the tendon itself mimic the changes that are found in the coracoacromial ligament. The bursal hypertrophy is a short staged phenomenon. Erosion of the bursa may leave a few bands until central cross-striation wear away and the bursal wall hypertrophies.

Continued impingement against the acromion, AC joint, clavicle and coracoacromial ligament leads to a hyperemic blush on the rotator cuff. The parallel, wavy, collagen-bundle structure is lost, there is an edematous change between these fibers, collagen necrosis and even focal calcification. Cellularity is diminished and there is very little evidence of repair. ACJ arthritis or coracoacromial ligament bony traction spur formation intensifies impingment.

Muscles must be balanced to effectively contain shoulder. If internal and external rotation strength is lost the humeral head is not depressed properly and this may cause superior migration allowing further wear of superior capsular structures. As the supraspinatus and biceps tendon wear, the humeral head rides higher. With the erosion progressing into the short depressors, the subscapularis, infraspinatus and teres minor may lose their depressor function. Because of angular change, they may start working as elevators, further accentuating the process and leading to end-stage impingement, wearing all the way through the supraspinatus, and allowing the humeral head to articulate with the acromion. As the humeral head migrates superiorly it loses its instant center of rotation, the deltoid becomes a less effective elevator and more of compressor, and wear countinues. In this situation, the scapulohumeral imbalance, if present, would further precipitate the disruption.

The cuff may finally wear through. Codman (1934) pointed out that rotator cuff tears can start from a rim rent.

Classification of rotator cuff impingement has been best described by Neer (1983), who subdivided rotator cuff tendinitis or impingement into three stages. Stage 1 is reversible edema and hemorrhage of the rotator cuff but should also include inflammation of the serosal and peripheral bursa that commonly occurs in patients under 25 years of age. This can be considered a subacute stage, because many athletes will ignore it. Stage 2 fibrosis and tendinitis occurring in patients from 25 to 40 years of age, is the usual status at initial clinical presentation. The bursa is no longer inflamed, and fibrotic changes may have already occurred within the bursa and the rotator cuff near the greater turberosity. Stage 3 tendinitis commonly occurs after age 40 and implies structural changes including bony changes and tendon ruptures, chronicity.

Further subdivision is necessary because structural cause must be identified in order to suggest the proper conservative or surgical method of treatment. Stage 3, or chronic tendinitis of the rotator cuff is a progressive phenomenon. At this stage, the factors that lead to progressive rotator cuff trauma may be clumped into three groups: group A-factors above the cuff, group B-factors below the cuff and group C-factors central to the cuff. These groups are interrelated, and it is often difficult to separate cause or effect within these groups because they overlap.

In group A, factors above the cuff, the coracoacromial arch and subacromial bursa are affected. The acromion may protrude on the cuff and bursa, causing erosion from development of traction spurs (within the anterior deltoid, within the lateral deltoid, or at the origin at the coracoacromial ligament) or central erosion caused by shape change due to superior migration of the humeral head combined with hypertrophy of anterior acromial bone. This hypertrophy may in fact be a braking mechanism that develops in an attempt to minimize anterior subluxation at the glenohumeral joint. The acromion helps to contain the humeral head in its socket, although this function may be lost from the effects of a nonfused apophysis, an apophyseal line loosened post trauma, or continued superior pressure from a loose glenohumeral joint. A ridge forms at the posterior aspect of the nonfused apophysis, which can also cause impingement. Fractures of the acromion or coracoid as well as degenerative arthritis and inferior spurring at the AC joint can cause encroachment into the supraspinatus outlet. With continuous inferior pressure due to loss of humeral head depression the acromion loses its containment ability, thus allowing further superior migration of the head and erosion of the cuff.

The serosal walls of the bursa invaginate the acromion, grow into trabecular interstices, develop a fibrocartilage layer that thickens the acromion, and allow further erosion into the cuff. A few fibrous bands snap as the althlete elevates his arm. In respones the impingement by rotation of the scapula, further wear at the chronic stage it becomes more fibrotic, especially peripherally, which significantly interferes with its sliding function. Again, normal biomechanical shoulder motion is disrupted. Thickening or fibrosis of the bursa and edema of the injured rotator cuff put pressure on the coracoid. These bony changes are even more traumatic to the cuff and further accelerate disease. Fibrosis of the burse is common in diabetics even if they are athletic.

Subcoracoid impingement occurs when the subscapularis is injured or partially thinned specifically when there is synovitis or contracture at the posterior capsule, which pulls, with a lax superoglenohumeral ligament or an anterior joint capsule with an enlarged interval defect (common in glenohumeral subluxation); this allows preferential superoanterior shifting of the humeral head, jamming it into the coracoid. Pain radiating down the medial aspect of the upper arm is characteristic of impingement against the coracoid and conjoined tendon. The cycle continues as impingement causes further erosion of the superior subscapularis fibers.

In group B factor below the cuff either damage to the superior suspension mechanism (associated with pitching or athletic trauma enlarging the rotator interval), stretching the coracohumeral ligament and damaging the biceps stabilizing mechanism, or glenohumeral laxity (which can eventually stretch out the superior capsule) leads to wear of the rotator cuff. Here, the initial partial tears are internal. The biceps and associated coracohumeral stabilizing ligaments are unable to stabilize the top of the joint when there is either posterior contracture of the capsule, anterior laxity of the superoglenohumeral mechanism, or failure of the supraspinatus or infraspinatus to depress the humeral head.

This increased motion at the top of the joint leads to microinstability, and supraspinatus insertional attrition near the greater tuberosity that tends to propagate with time. Breakdown in this area is also accelerated by glenohumeral arthritis.

Objects within the joint, such as a stub of a biceps tendon, a loose body, or a fragment of a torn labrum, can shift the humeral head out of the socket just slightly, causing functional subluxation and an abnormal pull at the supraspinatus insertion, which shifts the humeral head toward the subcoracoid impingement. Wobble at the top of the joint leads to erosion into superior subscapularis fibers and impaction against the coracoid and to associated vascular changes of the humeral head.

Group C includes changes of the rotator cuff itself. Early edema within the cuff will increase friction between the acromion and humeral head. Partial tearing either superficial or deep may cause a catching sensation that will change the normal smooth mechanics in activities such as throwing or lifting and altered mechanics may perpetuate the impingement process. In growth of scar in the healing process may inhibit motion, which leads to selective atrophy of the muscle fibers that are no longer exercised through their full range. Further exercised through their full range, thus further altering mechanics and leading to further impingement. Interstitial tearing within the cuff, even without external or internal partial erosion can lead to fusiform dilation that interfered with smooth motion. When the sliding motion of the supraspinatus under the acromion is lost, secondary muscles may be over used, leading to breakdown of other structures, the best example being periscapular muscle spasm. Calcific changes due to necrosis of the cuff near the greater tuberosity, traction spurring of the greater tuberosity, and avulsion fractures near the greater tuberosity insertion all interfere with normal mechanics and lead to impingement and subsequent wear of the cuff. A tear may lead with a fibrotic component that may be thickened and prone to further erosion. The long biceps tendon can be considered part of the rotator cuff. Its rupture can lead to loss of humeral head depression, allowing further superior migration of the humeral head and further wear of the remainder of the cuff.

NATURAL HISTORY

If rotator cuffs strain is left untreated, a vicious cycle is set up: Either calcific changes occur at tendinous or ligamentous insertions, which are abrasive and allow rotator cuff wear or muscle atrophy leading to stiffness, particularly in the back of the shoulder, which can progress to further weakness, further subluxation and stretching of the joint capsule. Although impingement in athletes can occur on its own, more commonly, it is a result of subluxation allowing the humeral head to slide forward and hit the acromion. Weakness of surrounding muscles and progressive superior migration lead to additional stretching of the capsule, which in turn, allows progressive impingement. Abnormal wear against the acromion transfers to the AC joint and can cause breakdown there as well. Ofcourse, previous trauma to the AC joint could lead to arthritis and cause wears into the rotator cuff, thus starting the cycle in reverse. Regardless, the end stage seems to be subluxation of the glenohumeral joint, erosion of the rotator cuff, and breakdown of the AC joint. This triad degeneration can be initiated by repetitive overhead use, common in swimming and pitching; and commonly by improper body mechanics or by attempting activity that the shoulder is not prepared for.

CLINICAL FEATURES

In early clinical presentation, the athlete complains of vague pain deep within the shoulder after athletic activity often described as a "toothache" type of pain. This pain is most pronounced in the overhead position, for example, at the point of releasing the baseball in throwing or when the hand touches the water in swimming. If the athlete attempts to bear the pain, it may eventually affect his or her ability to participate in the sport. When the athlete states that it feels as if the arm is "going dead" in addition to pain, weakness, snapping, or stiffness, it indicates subluxation.

HISTORY

In diagnosing chronic rotator cuff injury patient's history is important. The spectrum of complaints corresponds fairly well to the amount of tissue damage. Pain is present in throwing action mainly. The condition may be annoying, i.e. pain the day after sport activity with no loss of function it may decrease by aspirin, or it may have led to progressive inability to use the arm for functional activity. The patient may state that the pain had been annoying for some time, may have responded to cortisone injections or rest, yet continued to worsen over time. The patient may relate an episode when something subsequently "popped within the shoulder" while swinging a bat, sliding into base, or swing a racquet. There may have been pain before, but he or she is no longer able to lift the arm. The dull pain after activity may have progressed to night pain or constant pain when attempting to lift the arm or with overhead activity, implicating propagation of the original tear. Not all full-thickness tears can be attributed to propagation of a smaller tear. Clinically acute trauma can cause tearing, popping and immediate inability to lift the arm.

PHYSICAL EXAMINATION

On physical examination there may be point tenderness in the interval between the acromion and coracoid process or near the greater tuberosity, and the pain may worsen with forward flexion and internal rotation. In pure rotator cuff tendinitis, raising the arm in palm-down abduction may be painful between 80° and 120°, which allows the greater tuberosity to impinge against the acromoin. Turning the hand over in palm-up abduction is more painful, subluxation of the glenohumeral joint is most likely the etiology of the impingement and should be treated primarily rather than the impingement.

Mid range abduction is the key to assessment. Pain in the 60° to 100° range with the palm-down is relieved with the palm-up, indicates primary rotator cuff tenditis. Inability to abduct more than 40° hiking the shoulder to produce this scapulothoracic abduction, implicates a full-thickness rotator cuff tear, subdeltoid fibrosis or soft tissue catching within the glenohumeral joint. Capsulitis occurs in the healing process of even a partial-thickness tear. There is usually a loss of more motion in the termination of abduction of forward flexion in the 30° to 40° range, or of 4 to 12 vertebrae of internal rotation. There may even be an inability to break the plane of the body when testing internal rotation behind the back.

Even though the supraspinatus is the most commonly strained muscle in the humeral body, it heals most of the time. Even a cause, a blockage of some motion or contracture about the capsule, which most commonly leads to posterior shoulder pain. There may be tenderness over the A/C joint that is made worse with horizontal flexion, but hyper-abduction is often difficult to assess with motion blocked in the upper range. Supraspinatus testing in functional abduction thumb-down against resistance demonstrates no weakness early on, but as pathology progresses resistance is easily overcome.

Fine crepitation may be felt when rotating the shoulder, which correlates with bursal sclerosis, inflammation, intra-articular labral interposition, or bands of adhesions within the subacromial bursa. Generalized grinding at 90° of abduction with internal rotation may be due to wear of the acromion against the roughened cuff and may occur in a pure impingement phenomenon. Testing in functional abduction in line with the scapula, thumb toward the floor pushing up against resistance (Empty can test), may cause pain, the patient may complain of a toothache-like pain near the deltoid insertion as the presenting symptom.

Pain with resisted palm-down 90° abduction indicates impingement. Pain with the palm up shows instability. Lateral displacement of the affected side scapula, posterior capsule tightness and resisted isometric tests of rotator cuff muscles form an important part of assessment.

RADIOGRAPHIC ASSESSMENT IN EARLY TENDINITIS

A four-view X-ray study is useful to check for underlying A/C joint arthritis (which may cause or contribute to impingement or wear into the rotator cuff) to check for subluxation signs, and to look for inferior acromial architectural changes common with impingement. Supraspinatus insertional sclerosis, originally described by Dodman (1934), is sign of traction at the greater tuberosity and of inflammation leading to subacromial trabecular absorption of bone. Small spurs on the coracoid process or greater tuberosity, or calcification of the coracoacromial ligament may be seen in midsubstance or at the acromial insertion. Erosion into the acromion or small spur formation, particularly on the AP film angled down 15° may indicate a deltoid traction spur or a density under the acromion associated with traction hypertrophy at the origin of the coracoacromial ligament. Calcific tendinitis in the supraspinatus is due to the impingement phenomenon and due to localized necrosis that further cuff degeneration.

The arthrogram tells definitely whether there is partial-thickness intra-articular or full-thickness rotation cuff tear. Depending on the radiologist's skill, diagnosis of a large full-thickness tear is accurate 95 to 98% of the time. It is key to determine whether or not a full-thickness tear is distracted. Partial-thickness intra-articular tears, however, are less defined, and the superficial erosion is usually missed unless a bursogram is done. Changes within the biceps tendon and irregularities on the cuff can be seen on an arthrogram, giving evidence of chronicity.

A CT-arthrogram is very useful in early stages of the disease when internal partial-thickness tears and concrurrent subluxation can be documented with increased joint volume and labral pathology.

A bone scans help to document early inflammatory arthritis change within the A/C joint or glenohumeral joint degeneration associated with cuff pathology. It can show synovitis but is not a very specific test. An MRI, on the other hand, can help to identify edematous change within tendon, fibrotic replacement of tendon, subacromial spurs, arthritic changes that cause indentation of the rotator cuff, arthritic change within the A/C joint glenohumeral joint, and even avascular necrosis of the humeral head.

DIFFERENTIAL DIAGNOSIS

Stiffness, arthritis and referred pain, primarily of neurologic origin can lead to similar symptoms and confuse diagnosis. Because effective treatment is found on accurate diagnosis, it is important to differentiate wear of the rotator cuff from other causes of symptoms in order to suggest effective management.

AC joint arthritis: It may cause pain in the shoulder as either an isolated phenomenon or from erosion into the cuff; a 15° angled-up AP film can help define involvement. History of previous trauma to the A/C joint is important.

Bone scan can be but is not often helpful in differential diagnosis. Arthrography can be helpful. Marcaine or xylocaine can help define whether symptoms arise primary from A/C joint pathology.

Calcific tendinitis: Calcific tendinitis, although within the spectrum of rotator cuff disease, can be evident on X-ray.

Instability

The most important factor to assess in differential diagnosis is the stability of the glenohumeral joint. The patient with a positive impingement test as well as a positive apprehension sign that is minimized by anterior pressure on the shoulder.

Triad Degeneration

Injury leads to disuse and associated decrease in strength. With weaknesses, comes muscle imbalance and progressive wear of the rotator cuff so that it does not slide as well under the acromion.

When A/C joint breakdown has also occurred it must also be addressed. Loss of motion particularly reverse extension or horizontal extension to the 90° abduction appoint seriously compromise the ability of the muscles about the shoulder to depress the humeral head due to loss of muscular integration or balance.

Arthritis in either the glenohumeral or the A/C joint can minimize motion and produce findings similar to impingement such as grinding throughout the range of motion in horizontal flexion. Apprehension and hyperabduction testing for the glenohumeral and A/C joints, respectively should be done.

Advanced Cuff Disease

Although a full-thickness rotator cuff tear is a part of the spectrum of injury, it is treated much differently than early inflammatory tendinitis. Surgical intervention is more likely to be considered for the full-thickness tear. Ultrasound, arthrography, or arthroscopy can help in differential diagnosis. Isolated biceps tendinitis is extremely rare but can have similar symptoms, and testing palm-up forward flexion against resistance may help define this entity when found painful.

Reflex Sympathetic Dystrophy

It is important to rule out reflex sympathetic dystrophy syndrome (RSDS). Diminishing use of the arm can minimize muscular pumping action to return blood to the heart. Pooling of blood in the extremity can lead to motion of the skin and edema in the digits, as well as temperature change and sensitivity to weather, which are the hallmarks of reflex sympathetic dystrophy syndrome. If diagnosis of RSDS is suspected, a triphase bone scan that finds a defined blush on the early phase is 98% effective for confirmation.

MANAGEMENT

When a patient with cuff failure is being examined, he or she often reports persistent discomfort, especially with elevation, or abduction and external rotation. The patient usually experiences night pain, inability to lie on the shoulder, weakness, joint noise, and diminishing function. On physical examination crepitus, muscular weakness of the external rotation and abductors, shoulder muscular atrophy, and diminished active motion may be noted. Specific special tests, discussed earlier, may be beneficial. Imaging evaluation tests such as radiography, arthrography, CT scans, and MRI may be used to confirm the diagnosis. The differentiation from rotator cuff tendinitis and rotator cuff tears may be accomplished through the previously mentioned imaging studies or through direct visual inspection (arthroscopy). In addition, care must be taken in the examination process to differentiate cuff tears from other causes of shoulder pain and weakness such as cervical spondylosis, suprascapular neuropathy, scapular pathologies, glenohumeral joint arthritis, acromioclavicular joint arthritis, and adhesive capsulitis.

The treatment of documented cuff tears varies on the degree of disability exhibited by the patient. A nonoperative treatment approach should be attempted prior to any surgical repair. The goals of the rehabilitation program are to enhance the strength of the surrounding musculature, enhance the force couples of the glenohumeral joint to dynamically stabilized the joint, and eliminate stress on the injured cuff tissues. The challenge is to enhance the efficiency of the surrounding muscles to prevent the humeral head from migrating superiorly. Takagishi reported that 44% patients with a documented cuff tear responded well to nonoperative treatment. If the symptoms of pain and dysfunction persist, then surgical repair may become necessary.

In managing impingement it is important to first rule out subluxation. Ideally, subluxation is treated first, and the secondary impingement should diminish as the shoulder becomes more stable. If there is significant wearing onto the cuff or concurrent A/C joint arthritis, such factors may need to be dealt with as well if surgery is indicated. Horizontal flexion, hyperabduction, and reverse extension stretching for the A/C joint can help regain the motion necessary to strengthen the internal and external rotators that depress the humeral head and minimize impingement.

In the early stages most often the athlete will present with early impingement symptoms. In these cases conservative management is most appropriate and usually effective. As disease progresses and the injury is major (partial and complete tears) arthroscopic intervention may be considered.

CONSERVATIVE MANAGEMENT

In primary impingement, inflammatory medications are useful to alleviate the symptoms. In swimmers and throwers, if they are diagnosed early in the course of disease, respond well to rest, nonsteroidal inflammatory medication, and therapeutic strengthening. Modalities such as ice before and after activity, decreasing activity to about half the practice level at which symptoms occurred, and stretching and then strengthening while progressively increasing activity as symptoms diminish are usually effective. Eccentric muscle strengthening is often best tolerated in early impingement rehabilitation.

In conservative management of the acute stage, RICE forms an important part of the treatment. Ice is widely used in the treatment of recent injuries or in acute or irritated forms of the chronic conditions. During this time, the inflammatory changes are in an exaggerated form in the tissues. There is exudation of plasma into the tissue with a local edema and vasodilatation. This distorts the tissue, stimulates pain nerve endings. Local harmones likes histamine also produce the pain. Cooling will diminish the rate of edema and the production of irritants. Pain can be alleviated by the application of cold by the reduction of edema and decreased release of pain-inducing irritants. Ice directly affects the conduction of pain receptors and neurons, reducing the velocity and number of impulses. It is evident that this latter effect would only occur in the skin and only if the temperature is much reduced. It is unlikely that the unmyelinated C-fibers would be affected since they have been shown to continue to conduct at very low temperatures. The thinly myelinated A-delta fibers which carry well-delineated 'fast' skin pain would be more susceptible. However, the pain due to tissue injury would be carried by fibers and this is the pain that is usually being treated. Here ice can be given in the form of ice-massage or cold packs (for 10 minutes).

Relative Rest

Rest is to be given to the shoulder accrording to the severity of the condition. One must avoid the movements and activities that reproduce or aggravate the pain. The other joints of the upper limb and body can be exercised. Rest allows healing by reducing the inflammation. Rest, elevation and compression reduce the edema and promote healing in the earliest stages. Pulsed high frequency electromagnetic energy also helps in the healing of the injured cuff. The electric field produces currents in the tissue which themselves cause magnetic fields and similarly, as already pointed out, the magnetic field passing through the tissues will cause eddy currents, i.e. an electric field. Electromagnetic energy 'stirs' ions, molecules, membranes and perhaps cells thus speeding up phagocytic activity, enzymatic activity, transport across membranes and so forth. This would account for the evident acceleration of inflammatory and healing processes.

The activities of all cells are related to their ionic environment. There is a characteristic potential difference across all cell membranes and muscle tissue; the outside of the membrane is maintained electrically positive to the inside. Some depolarization of the cell membrane is often associated with cell dysfunction and electrical potential develops during wound with cell dysfunction and electrical potential is also involved in the control of growth, development and repair. It has been proposed that the electromagnetic field could influence the flow of ions through the membrane and therefore restore the normal cell potential in some damaged cells.

T Song (1989) postulated that cells are capable of absorbing energy from oscillating electrical fields of defined frequencies (frequency windows) and amplitudes, and making use of this energy for chemical work (Segal 1989), an increase in Na+ influx was produced in one direction, and a reduction in the other. When the epithelium rotated through 180° the effect was reversed.

An increase in the number and activity of cells in the injured region, reabsorption of hematoma, reduced inflammation, reduced swelling, increased rate of fibrin deposition and orientation, increased collagen deposition and organization, increased nerve growth and repair.

A dosage of 40–65 ms, 400–600 pps, 20 min. can be given 1 time a day. Slowly as acute stage subsides, isometric exercises are given and supraspinatus initiation exercise is begun. It is very important to see that muscle strength is not lost by giving excess and unwanted rest to the part.

Ultrasound therapy: If local temperature is raised to between 40 and 45°C, hyperemia will result (Lehmann and Guy, 1972). Temperatures above 45°C are destructive. To achieve a useful therapeutic effect the tissue temperature has to be maintained between these values for at least 5 min (Lehman and delLateur, 1982). Heating fibrous tissue structures such as joint capsules, ligaments, tendons and scar tissue structures can cause a temporary increase in their extensibility, and hence a decrease in joint stiffness. The advantage of using ultrasound to achieve this healing is due to the preferential heating of collagen tissue and to the effective penetration of this energy to deeply placed structures. However, ultrasound-absorbing structure can prevent the treatment reaching deeply placed target tissue if they intervene in the path of the sonic beam (Dyson, 1987). Mild heating can also have the effect of reducing pain and muscle spasm and promoting healing processes. Kramer (1987), investigating the increase in conduction velocity in motor and sensory nerves following therapeutic ultrasound, concluded that this was likely to be related to the heating effect of ultrasound.

Additionally, as a result of either type of cavitation there is a localized, unidirectional fluid movement around the vibrating bubble. These very small fluid movements around cells are called microstreaming and are believed to play a significant role in the therapeutic effect of ultrasound (Dyson, 1987). Such streaming is said to affect the permeability of cell membranes where it is particularly marked. Its effect is to alter the rate of diffusion of ions across the membrane, for example calcium which, as a second messenger, may result in the stimulation of repair processes and sodium which possibly alters electrical activity in nerves, and could, therefore, be involved in pain relief.

Acute Stage

The effects of stable cavitation and accousting steaming appear to increase calcium across the cell membrane. This, in turn, causes mast cell degranulation with the release of histamine and other factors. In this way, ultrasound has the potential to accelerate normal resolution of inflammation providing that the inflammatory stimulus is removed (Dyson, 1987). This acceleration could also be due to the gentle agitation of the tissue fluid which may increase the rate of phagocytosis and the movement of particles and cells (Elvans, 1980).

Granulation Stage

This begins approximately 3 days after injury and is the stage at which the connective tissue framework is laid down by fibroblast for the new blood vessels. During repair, fibroblasts may be stimulated to produce more collagen; it has been shown that ultrasound can promote collagen synthesis (Harvey et al. 1975). This is thought to be due to increased cell membrane permeability, caused by ultrasound, allowing the entry of calcium ions which control cellular activity (Dyson, 1987). Not only is more collagen formed but it is also of greater tensile strength after ultrasound treatment.

Ultrasound is also believed to encourage the growth of new capillaries in chronic ischemic tissue and the same could happen during repair of soft tissues after injury (Dyson, 1987). The enhanced released of growth factors from macrophages following exposure to therapeutic ultrasound has also been observed (Young, 1988).

Ultrasound is considered to improve the extensibility of mature collagen such as is found in scar tissue (Lehman and deLateur, 1982). This is believed to occur by promoting the reorientation of the fibers (remodeling) which leads to greater elasticity without loss of strength.

Direct contact application can be given with arm in a position where the tendons are most superficial, e.g: internal rotation for the tendons attached on greater tubercle. 1 MHZ head is used with an intensity of 0.8 to 1 wtt/cm^2 for 4-5 minutes.

DEEP TRANSVERSE FRICTION MASSAGE

The mobilization of tissues by forming thumb or index finger and the skin as one unit moving over the selected tissue below the skin helps in increasing the local circulation, re-alignment of the healing fibers or scar in a normal way, improves the extensibility and healing of the sensory stimulus also gives an efficient mode to help healing and reduce pain.

EXERCISES

Rehabilitation of throwing athlete can be divided into 4 components—stretching, strengthening, postural correction and a progressive throwing program.

Initially dynamic stability is developed during the stability and controlled mobility producers in close chain activities. Normally stability of the scapulothoracic and glenohumeral joint encompasses the ability to maintain proper alignment during open and closed chain activities in varying ranges with different biomechanical stresses against isometric resistive forces. Controlled mobility implies normal scapulohumeral rhythm during weight shifting in weight bearing postures. Both stability and controlled mobility are components of proximal dynamic stability and skilled movement.

Scapular stability is initially developed by performing low-intensity isometric contractions, first in shortened ranges and then in more lengthened ranges. The isometric contractions improve muscle's automatic responses by enhancing the proprioceptive sensitivity of the muscle spindle.

D1 flexion (flexion, adduction and external rotation) then D2 flexion (flexion, abduction and external rotation) with emphasis on scapula depression and adduction and shoulder internal and external rotation form a part of the initial treatment.

This sequence is chosen to gradually increase the challenge on rotator cuff while maintaining proper relation of humeral head in glenoid and avoid movements causing impingement.

In chair sitting position, hand on the couch at side of body, alternating isometrics and rhythmic stabilization can be done. It may progress to a quadrupled position (45-60° of flexion) for the same and then in standing position hands on wall (60 to 120° flexion). This is useful by the impingement in activity of trapezius, rhomboids, serratus, rotator cuff and deltoid to increase the proximal stability. Abnormal responses include excessive scapular abduction, elevation on thorax or flickering of the muscles around the shoulder. These responses indicate that the intensity of body weight is too great or that the maintenance of the posture is too long. The exercises can be progressed by weight shifting and increasing the weight on affected side. The range and direction of proximal motion and the amount of weight bearing resistance can be varied. The direction of rocking may progress from D1 flexion to D2 flexion.

Coordinated movement between scapular shoulder muscles while maintaining and performing more biomechanically challenging activities is indicative of proximal dynamic stability. Within the scapula, this level of control requires a "balance" between the adductor and abductors and between the elevator and depressors maintain a mid-range position as body weight and stretch increases the challenge to stabilize. In the shoulder a balance of forces between the rotator cuff and the extrinsic muscles is required. Dynamic stability of proximal muscles is essential for effective scapulohumeral rhythm. The normal timing of skilled movement is developed as the stability, controlled mobility and static-dynamic stages are performed in the sequence of weight bearing postures. Abnormal scapular movements include lifting of the scapula off the thorax (serratus anterior weakness), upward tilt of the inferior angle (lower trapezius weakness), excess abduction into scapula (tight posterior capsule, weakness of middle trapezius and rhomboids).

Progression of activities can be done by resistance also. Open chain activities follow the weight bearing exercises.

D1 flexion (scapular protraction, shoulder flexion adduction, external rotation using serratus, anterior deltoid and rotators) to D1 extension (scapular retraction, shoulder extension, abduction and internal rotation using rhomboids, posterior deltoid and rotator cuff) and D2 flexion (scapular elevation, shoulder flexion, abduction, external rotation using trapezius, middle deltoid and rotator cuff to D2 extension (scapular depression, shoulder extension, abduction and internal rotation using pectoralis minor, pectoralis major and rotator cuff) can be included gradually.

All patients presenting with impingement or rotator cuff tendinitis should be started on a rehabilitation program. Rehabilitation of an athlete's shoulder can be divided into four phases: rest, stretching, strengthening followed by a progressive throwing program.

Rest involves restriction from the aggravating activity. This should be combined with passive range of motion exrcises to maintain flexibility. Anti-inflammatory medication, ice, and gentle message can be added to expedite the inflammatory phase. In competitive athletes, it is important to maintain cardiovascular fitness during the rest period. Lower extremity exercises and conditioning which does not affect the shoulder should be performed.

Once the shoulder is pain-free, stretching excercises can be added. Stretching should focus on returning to full range of motion, especially internal and external rotation. Throwers typically have greater external rotation and less internal rotation. The stretching program must not aggravate a pathologic condition, particularly, anterior instability. Capsular tightness is not uncommon in a sore overused shoulder. Increased posterior capsular tightness can result in anterior translation and worsen a secondary impingement. It can also limit internal rotation, leading to increased scapular excursion in the follow-through, medial scapular pain, and medial scapular muscle fatigue. The goal of a stretching program is to have a balanced range of motion without pain or stiffness in any position. Any subtle loss of motion can result in major imbalance.

After a full pain-free range of motion has been achieved, a strengthening program can be initiated. The strengthening program initially focuses on the dynamic stabilizers of the glenohumeral joint, the rotator cuff. These are the most important muscles for proper shoulder function. A program of rotator cuff and scapulohumeral excercises that involve a Theraband, light hand weights, and painless effort early in the program. Light weights and high repetitions are the rule. Specific internal rotation excercises are introduced later on in the program, because of the dominance of these muscles over the external rotators. Exercises with the elbow extended through a vertical plane in internal rotation can exacerbate impingement pathology and are avoided. If pain develops, the exercises are discontinued and the patient is reevaluated. Aerobic activities not involving the shoulder may be performed.

The program should not overlook the scapular rotators. These muscles are extremely important to correct throwing mechanics and the stability of the joint during the throwing process. Stretching and strengthening of the serratus anterior, trapezius, and medial scapular muscles should be included in the shoulder program.

In a study by Moseley et al., the scapular rotator muscles examined by EMG analysis during a shoulder rehabilitation program. Four exercises (scapular plane elevation, row push-up plus, and press up) were considered key to strengthening of these muscles.

The anterior deltoid has five exercises that met the criterion. The leading exercises are elevation of the arm in the scapular plane (scaption) with the arm internally rotated. This has a peak activity of 72% MMT. The next highest qualifiers are scaption in external rotation and flexion both the peak activities in the fourth concentric arcs of 71% and 69% MMT respectively, and durations of 30% and 31%. Military press and abduction both have of 62% MMT in the second and fourth concentric arcs, respectively, and duration of 50% and 31%.

Scaption in internal rotation is also the top exercise for the middle deltoid, with a peak of 83% MMT during the fourth concentric arc and duration of 70%. Horizontal abduction in internal rotation, horizontal abduction in external rotation, and flexion are next height with peak activities in the fourth concentric arcs of 80%, 79%, and 73% MMT and duration of 38%, 57%, and 31%, respectively. Scaption in external rotation, rowing and military press and are peaks of 72% MMT in the fourth concentric arc, and duration of 58%, 43% and 38% respectively, abduction 64% MMT in the fourth concentric arc and a duration of 31%. Deceleration has a 58% peak MMT in the third concentric arc of motion and a 27% duration.

The leading exercises for the posterior deltoid are horizontal abduction both with the arm in internal (peak of 93% MMT) and external rotation (peak of 92% MMT) during the fourth concentric arc and durations of 63% and 57% respectively. Rowing is third with a peak of 88% MMT in the fourth concentric arc and a duration of 57%. External rotation display a peak of 64% MMT at the third concentric arc and a 43% duration. A peak activity of 63% MMT in the third concentric arc was noted deceleration, having duration of 27%.

The supraspinatus has four exercises that meet the criterion. The top exercise was military press, which had a peak activity of 80% MMT at the first concentric arc and duration of 50%. Scaption with internal rotation is coined with a peak value of 74% MMT at the fourth concentric arc and duration of 40%. Flexion has a peak fourth concentric arc of 67% MMT and a duration of 31%. Scaption with external rotation was peak of 64% MMT and duration of 25%.

The subscapularis has exercises meeting the initial criterion. Therefore, the qualifying criterion is decreased to two arcs of motion over 50% MMT. At this level only one exercise, scaption with internal rotation, qualified. The peak activity is 62% MMT seen at the fifth concentric arc with a duration of 22%. If the criterion is decreased to 40% MMT, there more exercises qualified, military press duration of 50%. Both flexion and abduction has peak in the fifth concentric arc of 52% and 50%

MMT, respectively and durations of 23%. Internal rotation has peak arc of 31% MMT.

The leading exercise for the infraspinatus is horizontal abduction with external rotation. This has a peak activity level of 88% MMT at the fourth concentric arc and a duration of 71%. External rotation has a peak of 85% MMT at the third concentric arc and a duration of 43%. Horizontal abduction in internal rotation has a peak of 74% MMT at the fourth concentric arc and a 38% duration. Five other exercises qualified for the infraspinatus are abduction, flexion, scaption in external rotation, deceleration, push up with hand together. The leading exercises for the teres minor are external rotation and horizontal abduction in external rotation, with peak activities of 80% and 74% MMT, respectively, and duration of 57%. The only other qulifier is horizontal abduction with internal rotation. It generates 68% MMT during the second concentric arc and had a duration of 43%.

The press up and push up with hands apart both qualify for the pectoralis major with peak arcs of 84% and 64% MMT. The durations are 75% and 50% respectively.

The press up was the only exercise to meet the criterion for the latissimus dorsi. This had 55% peak activity during the 1st second of isometric contraction and a duration of 50%.

Internal rotation, bench press, and horizontal adduction did not meet the qualifying criterion for any of the muscles.

Of the four exercises meeting the criterion for the supraspinatus (military press, both scaption maneuvers, and flexion) all are involved in humeral elevation).

Even though scaption demonstrated high EMG activity at elevation above 90°, such a level of elevation is not clinically recommended. Once the arm is elevated above 90° in the scapular plane, impingement can occur. Thus scaption above 90° is not recommended. Scaption can be done up to 90° with a heavier weight which would produce the enhanced muscle activity, or flexion can be selected as a more ideal exercise. Flexion involves a very similar pattern of muscle activity to scaption in internal rotation without risking impingement.

The sequential goals of rehabilitation are to (1) return to normal passive and active range of motion (2) re-establish synchrony of motion (3) increase strength and endurance in integrated muscle action, and (4) progressively return pitching.

Complete Shoulder Girdle motion

The goal of the flexibility program in a pitching shoulder is to obtain normal glenohumeral motion. Achieving normal glenohumeral and scapulothoracic motion is an absolute necessity before strengthening programs are begun. With normal glenohumeral motion, glenohumeral scapulothoracic musculature can interact and coordinate the forces which occur to all surroundings of the tissue structure of the shoulder. Without flexibility ill-advised strength programs will enhance abnormal movement patterns.

Pitchers who have significant tightness can obtain flexibility effectively through the use of proprioceptive neuromuscular facilitation technique (PNF). These techniques are extremely helpful in conditions where limitation of motion is a prime concern. PNF techniques are able to enhance relaxation of antagonistic muscle patterns and facilitate agonistic muscle activity. There are a variety of PNF techniques available.

To achieve flexibility in horizontal flexion, patient supine and stabilize the scapula as much as possible behind the thorax. A slow, sustained stretch is applied as the humerus is brought across the chest wall to gain glenohumeral horizontal flexion to either 45° or within the limits allowed by the chest wall.

To achieve an increased excursion of the combined abduction pattern, position the patient supine and stabilize the scapula at the edge of the thoracic wall. A slow, sustained passive stretch combined with the use of active neuromuscular facilitation techniques is applied to the arm in a downward direction toward the table.

Care should be taken not to exceed a range beyond the horizontal level of the table. Movement beyond the horizontal may cause the anterior capsule of the shoulder to be stretched too far, precipitating a local inflammatory response, increasing joint laxity, or leading to an anterior labral tear. Bicipital tendinitis may also result from excessive motion in this pattern.

Proper patterning muscle action is an important prerequisite to a healthy pitching shoulder. A sequence of shoulder abduction, horizontal extension, and external rotation occurs during the cocking phase. If a pitcher is unable to perform this sequence in an upright position, symmetrically, without any indication of weakness or lack of scapular stabilization, it is wise to use the sequence of active abduction, horizontal extension, and external rotation as an exercise. Pitchers should practice this pattern at least twice per day for 25 repetitions each. Concentration should be on scapular stabilization and bilateral symmetrical motion. Scapulohumeral rhythm is difficult to accomplish for a pitcher with marked shoulder weakness. As flexibility, strength, and scapular stabilization improve, lateral scapular migration will decrease. Proper attention given to the pattern of muscle action will ensure a stable shoulder during the entire pitching sequence.

PROGRESSIVE RESISTANCE EXERCISES

Pitching necessitates complete dynamic muscular balance around the shoulder. Muscular balance in a dynamic sense is essential. For a minor muscle imbalance during throwing will result in a pattern of muscle substitution which leads to further imbalance. Of particular importance, when planning a strengthening program for the pitching shoulder are muscles acting both the glenohumeral and scapulothoracic joint. It is important not to start strengthening exercise until flexibility, synochrony of motion of the shoulder girdle complex, and distinct contractions in all shoulder musculature through a normal range have been achieved. Strengthening before the return of normal motion enhances abnormal patterns of movement, which subsequently lead to a cycle of strength/motion loss.

Initially a pitcher should complete the exercise regimen without any weight and progress at 1 to 2 pound increments once the exercise can be completed appropriately, i.e., without muscle substitution. The exercises are performed in a concentric eccentric manner with a slow concentric contraction followed by a slow eccentric contraction to the starting position. Eccentric contractions are important for the deceleration of the arm in the follow through phase (eccentric contractions). Frequent repetition, low weight (5 pounds maximum) exercises are recommended for restrengthening program. There is no need to exceed 5 pounds tend to precipitate a loss of muscular balance around the throwing shoulder. Three sets of the repetitions are a goal for each exercise.

PROGRESSIVE PITCHING

1. *Mirror throwing:* The pitcher with chronic shoulder discomfort frequently has not thrown with his normal motion for at least half a season and usually longer. When flexibility has been restored, muscle integration attained, evident control of his shoulder during the patterns of the pitching motion achieved, practice of the pitching motion with light weight (1 pound) in the throwing hand can be initiated. The pitcher is instructed to use his normal pitching motion in front of a mirror, and be cognizant of each phase, particularly the exaggeration of the horizontal extension and external rotation of the cocking phase. By performing the act slowly, each muscle is conditioned in three specific activities (1) the posterior excursion of the throwing arm, (2) fixation of the shoulder girdle necessary to provide an eccentric resistance so that the shoulder might rotate about a fixed point, and (3) the smooth follow-through so that the stress of deceleration might be distributed among all soft tissue structures. This deceleration awareness exercise is an excellent method of conditioning the posterior shoulder musculature in the eccentric contraction necessary for enlarged deceleration forces of the follow through.
2. *Short distance throwing:* In combination with mirror throwing, the pitcher may begin to play catch with a ball for short distance of 20 to 30 feet and progress from periods of 5 minutes to 15 to 20 minutes daily.

3. *Long distance arc throwing:* When the pitcher is able to throw short distance for 20 to 30 minutes comfortably, long distance throwing can be initiated. The throw should be delivered to a partner on an arc. The pitcher should concentrate on proper mechanics and use total body motion while throwing.
4. *Form pitching:* This period is usually a minimum of 6 to 8 weeks after the start of a conditioning program for a shoulder with chronic discomfort.

   Progress towards a home program is done with a return to full activity when the strength deficit is less than 20% of the opposite shoulder or less than 20% of what is normal for the patient's height and weight, if there is too initial response to physical therapy at 6 weeks or if the patient is too uncomfortable, a CT-arthrogram is taken alone for the younger athlete, and include a bone scan for the older athelete because A/C joint arthritis may be some concern. CT-arthrography helps define a full-thickness tear of the rotator cuff or signs of labral damage that indicate subluxation.

Injection

It is important to avoid steroid injection in treatment of cuff disease. By decreasing inflammation, injection may minimize healing process, unravel collagen, and may contribute in effect to subsequent propagation of the tear in areas of fiber fatigue. Pain is a protective mechanism and if taken away and may not protect the athlete against the offending activity that can make the impingement worse. Kennedy and Willis (1976) injected steroid into healthy tendon and notice that it unraveled collagen and made the tissue more edematous; reorganization of the collagen took 6 or more weeks. If the pain response is diminished, it perhaps causes more damage. If a decision is made to use cortisone injection, it is important that the athlete understands that it leaves the muscle fibers at risk. Steroid injections should be used judiciously.

Shoulder biomechanics and proper technique of the sport must be assessed to help avoid future irritation of the rotator cuff. An exercise program recommended by the physician and therapist must be maintained.

When there is no response to conservative management, i.e. continued pain in spite of increased motion and strength with therapy, then surgery may be an option. Surgery must be avoided unless preceded by mobilization; operation on a stiff joint may lead to an even stiffer joint. Surgery consists of evaluation under anesthesia, manipulation to regain remaining lost motion, arthroscopic assessment, and perhaps either inferior arthroscopic acromioplasty or endoscopic debridement of arthritis or spurs at the A/C joint. Judgment should be made about what part of the acromion is offending the cuff and whether the coracoacromial ligament is involved.

Removing the weight and placing the arm through range of motion at the time of arthroscopic analysis to check where impingement occurs can aid in assessment by defining corresponding worn area of the acromion and cuff. The weight is returned to give clearance for surgery and the affected area of bone or soft tissue (bursal adherence to the undersurface of acromion or thickened bursa) is debrided. The weight is again removed, and if there is further impingement, then bone in the area of irritation is also debrided. This usually includes just the anterior rim of the acromion. However, if there is A/C joint arthritis a dome decompression at the undersurface of the joint or joint resection can be useful to remove impinging osteophytes and regain A/C joint motion. When the coracoacromial ligament is involved, cauterization is generally necessary to diminish bleeding, unless one of the fluid management systems is utilized.

Partial-thickness tears of the rotator cuff can be dealt with arthroscopically. The internal articular side tears are debrided to prevent irritation of the biceps tendon and catching within the joint. Loose, frayed material is not debrided to stimulate healing but to better assess whether there is a full-thickness tear. Debridement of intra-articular amplifying factors, such as labral tearing, frayed superior glenohumeral ligament tissue, and so on, can help minimize symptoms in rehabilitation.

The actual areas of impingement can be defined removing the weight at the time of arthroscopy. The undersurface of the acromion that directly contacts the edematous or worn part of the rotator cuff usually has a "crab meat" appearance. Debriding this acromial segment is all that is necessary to minimize symptoms. This is safely accomplished by keeping and working from the back of the A/C joint forward toward the front.

Subacromial bursal bands and thickening or fibrosis of the bursa that minimize the smooth lubricated motion of the cuff, if found, should be debrided. Smoothing of a flap near the eroded area of the cuff, debridement of acromial and clavicular spurs, and debridement of irregular bursal tissue can give smoother motion, which minimizes wear related pain in athletic activity, particularly in the recreational athlete. When discomfort is minimized, stretching, strengthening, and rehabilitation are more likely to be successful.

The majority of patients will have partial-thickness intra-articular or occasional extra-articular tear of the rotator cuff under previous impinging acromial or clavicular spurs. Even with a very small hole, most patients respond to arthroscopic debridement. They require conservative management consisting of strengthening and stretching but usually no additional surgical intervention. If additional surgery is required after passive motion is regained in therapy, then open repair decompression with or without a Mumford procedure or concurrent stabilization of the glenohumeral joint may be indicated as a second surgical stage. The mobilized tissue is easier to repair. Elimination of stiffness ensures a better post-surgical result.

If surgery is done, rehabilitation is mandatory first to regain motion and then strength. Mobilization helps to prevent recurrence of adhesions and fibrosis; internal and external rotation with the arm at the side and then use functional abduction exercises. Keeping the muscle balanced, exercise program is mandatory to help avoid recurrence of impingement.

If arthroscopic subacromial decompression is not sufficient to diminish symptoms, open reduction and internal fixation of the loose anterior acromial fragment can be consideration.

Management of chronic rotator cuff change depends on the extent of symptoms. Most patients who are treated for bursitis or "bicipital tendinitis" have in fact rotator cuff disease, which may be misdiagnosed. Treatment is geared first towards restoration of motion. Fibrosis or a partially "frozen" shoulder must be overcome in an effort to rehabilitate the shoulder. Once motion is regained then muscular strength can be worked on. It must be emphasized to the patient that the minor snapping caused by residual bands of scar tissue within the shoulder is of no considerable consequence unless it hurts.

Of prime importance is strengthening. If the humeral head depressors (even if the supraspinatus static depressor) are weak, preferential strengthening of the subscapularis and infraspinatus can hold the humeral head down slightly diminishing symptoms and minimize supraspinatus grinding. Strengthening of the deltoid, biceps, triceps, and periscapular stabizers can significantly minimize supraspinatus symptoms. Working on flexibility can help minimize subsequent propagation of tear.

When conservative management is not effective in alleviating the pain associated with partial or full-thickness cuff tear i.e. if there has been no improvement in active elevation of the arm after a complete tear (i.e. surrounding musculature does not compensate for the tear), surgery is indicated. Endoscopic bursal surgery is useful in resection of pathologic changes that lead to wearing of the rotator cuff.

Arthroscopic Mobilization

In treatment of chronic impingement, a two-stage surgical approach should be evaluated under anesthesia to regain motion. Concurrent glenohumeral arthroscopy allows treatment of amplifying factors such as labral sprains or slaps lesions. Arthroscopic debridement within the joint and assessment of the rotator cuff is then followed by bursoscopy of the subacromial space with acrominoplasty and resection of bursal and subdeltoid adhesions. Adhesion resection can increase mobility of the rotator cuff significantly. A second stage open cuff repair is often avoided due to the relief of pain from mobilization and debridement alone.

Open Exposure

With a large tear of significant wearing into the cuff under the A/C joint, a utility incision is most useful for open repair. This is an incision in line with the end of the clavicle across the acromion; the deep incision is in line with the skin incision but curves of the acromion down into the deltoid paralleling fiber arrangement. This wide exposure allows resection of the A/C joint and cuff repair or imbrication. With coexistent glenohumeral pathology a safer incision is used so that both conditions can be dealt with concurrently.

Cuff Imbrication

Significant erosion into the cuff thins the cuff and makes balancing and containing the humeral head more difficult. Bone and tissue protrusion into the supraspinatus outlet can cause a worn area in the rotator cuff. This uncreative area usually becomes less symptomatic after arthroscopic subacromial decompression, dome decompression of the A/C joint or endoscopic or open distal clavicle resection. Scarring in the healing process, however, may minimize motion and lead to the need for future physical therapy, manipulation under anesthesia, or arthroscopy debridement of the new scar. The worn area may not heal even if full motion is restored, in which case the patient may complain of a constant dull ache directly under the previously impingement A/C joint area that get worse with weather change, leading to the need for open repair of the ulcer. Surgical imbrication of the worn cuff may be necessary to restore a smooth surface to ride under the acromion so that scapulothoracic overuse can be minimized.

Cuff Repair

Repair of the hole in cuff is very effective in decreasing the pain that radiates to the root of the deltoid. In a younger individual the cuff may have been pulled of by acute trauma, and repair without decompression may be all that is necessary. If soft tissue or bony changes have developed, they must also be dealt with concurrently. This would mean appropriate acromioplasty (either anterior, medial, or lateral depending on the size of the spur), stabilization of a mesoacromial apophyseal nonunion (which uncommonly coexits with glenohumeral instability or superior impact injury), distal clavicectomy for A/C joint arthritis, tightening of the coracohumeral suspensory system, or capsular stabilization of the glenohumeral joint when appropriate.

A very small rotator cuff tear can be ignored if amplifying factors are removed in either an open or arthroscopic procedure. Arthroscopically assisted surgery has the potential of minimizing irritation of the deltoid muscle, which is important in rehabilitation. A very small hole can be usually ignored but is easily repaired through a miniarthrotomy incision, which is an extension of the anterolateral portal towards the A/C joint. A moderately sized hole of 1 to 3 cm, identified by arthrogram as non-displace or minimally displaced, can be repaired through a mini-arthrotomy.

Interscalene or regional block can yield enough pain relief to allow miniarthrotomy to be done as an outpatient procedure. Rather than the traditional method of making a trough, which needs significant advancement of tissue, merely abrading the greater tuberosity area, sinking a subcortical anchor, and bringing the rotator cuff to this freshened area can yield enough tissue to close a small or moderate size tear. The patient is immobilized for 4 weeks, pendulum exercises can be started the following day, and relief of pain from the chemical irritation of joint fluid leaking out of the hole is almost instantaneous.

A bolus of IV antibiotics is usually given in the outpatient center prior to discharge. Postoperative physiotherapy forms an important form of treatment, which includes strengthening exercises, pain relieving modalities and functional rehabilitation.

A larger hole, however, necessitates greater exposure, usually by stripping the deltoid from the acromion and distal clavicle, and is therefore more painful. The length of time for postoperative immobilization and initiation of pendulum exercises is usually the same as for an outpatient procedure. It may be extended by 2 weeks if there is some tension of the repair. The use of an abduction splint is no longer advocated, because a muscle healing in an abducted position most likely will rip as the arm is brought down to the side when the brace is removed.

Many "irreparable" rotator cuff tears can be repaired by subdeltoid adhesion resection and mobilization of tissue by endoscopic Mumford distal clavicectomy or dome decompression of inferior acromial spurs can be done. Removal of inferior acromial spurs can be done concurrently. If arthroscopic distal clavicle resection and inferior acromioplasty has been done, often a short 3-cm anterolateral incision, extending the anterolateral distally forms the edge of the acromion towards the A/C joint marking needle, is all that is needed for a short tear.

With repair, the transposed muscle may be pulled apart with early use or may no longer pull in the same direction, so that motion will be jeopardized. A large tear that cannot be easily closed should most likely be left alone to obtain the best functional result. For older individual, motion is more important than attempting to regain power. Golf and doubles tennis may be substituted for overhand throwing and weight training.

Irreparable Cuff Debridement

Although subdeltoid adhesion resection may change the situation, occasionally a massive tear may not be repairable, debridement of irregularities of the acromioclavicular joint, bursal edges, and so can decrease friction and minimize symptoms. These can be done arthroscopically or as open procedures. Transposing a tendon may alter the effective vector of its pull and even though some strength may be regained, a decreased amount of motion is usually associated. Trying to close a large defect may minimize function. A surprising number of elderly recreational athletes with large full thickness rotator cuff tears recover well with arthroscopic debridement. However, with adequate flexibility and strengthening from exercising the remaining tissue, very few of these athletes need open operative procedures. They tend to be slightly weaker than patients who have had cuff repair but they have motion which is ultimately more important.

Salvage Arthroplasty

Subacromial decompression, either open or arthroscopic, is most effective when there has been no superior upriding of the humeral head. Once the humeral head has button holed through the rotator cuff defect, which implies failure of the humeral head depressors, it is very difficult to decelerate the degenerative cycle. This leads to end-stage impingement disease in which the humeral head articulates with the acromion, coracoid or undersurface of the clavicle. The athlete may possibly have to give up active participation in athletics before this occurs, so the goal in treatment should be to avoid this stage. Salvage, pain relief, and return to daily activities, rather than return to athletic activity, become the goals.

Total joint arthroplasty is not effective in taking care of these problems, because the supraspinatus static depressor is no longer effective, the subscapularis active depressor is commonly stretched or frayed, and the teres minor and infraspinatus depressors are usually contracted. The best that can be done is to use a large hemiprosthesis of the humeral head of help regain an instant center and to help the deltoid and remaining muscles to function near their optimal length. Even in the end-stage impingement, subacromial decompression can be effective in pain relief, although it is much less predictable. Much depends on restraining the deltoid to elevate in lower range.

If the rotator cuff is strengthened in therapy primarily by exercising the supraspinatus and deltoid muscles, the imbalance of the internal and external rotators (common in subluxation) may get worse, and the patient will complain of more pain in therapy than before therapy, a condition also found with a functional subluxation, and work only on the inwardly rotated pendulum and Codman exercises, with the left shoulder clockwise and the right shoulder counter clockwise. Rotation in the opposite direction mimics the abducted, externally rotated apprehension maneuver and will make the patient feel more uncomfortable when subluxation is the underlying problem. In this situation, therapy is completely reversed, with internal rotation strengthening done first, progressing towards external rotation balancing, and then external rotation in functional elevation. Exercise the supraspinatus and medial deltoid elevator muscles only after the depressor muscles of the cuff (infraspinatus, subscapularis, and anterior and posterior deltoid) are stronger.

Arthroscopic surgical decompression may make the underlying subluxation worse by allowing further superior migration of the humeral head. Ideally, relief of secondary impingement symptoms will allow the patient to return to strengthening exercises to depress the humeral head and treat the primary glenohumeral instability problem. If therapy fails in this case, however, subsequent tightening of the shoulder capsule may be of some benefit. Even in an open, acromioplasty it is very important not to take out too much acromion, because the anterior acromial hook may have developed as a stabilizer to prevent anterior to posterior subluxation of the shoulder. Removal of the hook may unmask the underlying instability or make it worse, leading to need for open stabilization.

Tear Propagation

The injuries of rotator cuff become worse and propagate to become tears of more extent. Complications occur from treatment and from lack of treatment. A tear in the rotator cuff may propagate while the patient is in therapy, and the patient must be warned ahead of time that this is risk. Avoiding such propagation can be done by stretching, and exercises for humeral head depression. Too aggressive or unsupervised physical therapy or improper use of isokinetic testing equipment for therapy may lead to failure.

Misdiagnosis

Too generous an acromioplasty, either arthroscopic or open, can lead to further superior migration of the humeral head and accelerate degeneration process both within the glenohumeral space and of the rotator cuff. Failure to properly diagnose, that is, operating on a clinical rotator cuff tear when adhesive capsulitis, instability, cervical radiculopathy, or tumor is the actual cause, can also lead to failure of management.

COMPLICATIONS OF SURGERY

Neurologic Dysfunction

Fibrosis in retracted rotator cuff tissue may mean that function of the suprascapular nerve is closed; loss of supraspinatus and infraspinatus innervation may mean no return of motor function.

Loss of Motion

Presenting with pain and loss of motion, the athlete may expect both to recover after repair. With a massive tear, fiber orientation gets altered in an attempt to close the hole. Repair may limit joint fluid from leaking out and minimize pain. However, the change in orientation of fibers necessary to accomplish this means that muscles are now pulling in different directions from the way they were meant to; therefore, motion is compromised. The repaired tendon in a full-thickness tear is by no means a normal tendon. Even with stable fixation to a roughened bone through area (which is made to encourage healing), acromioplasty, subacromial decompression, and adequate immobilization, the advanced tissue may not hold, and failure of the operative repair is a possibility.

Failed Tendon Repair

The main complication of rotator cuff repair is cuff failure. This is due to many factors: the tissue paper-like cuff often found at time of repair, reorientation of remaining cuff fibers in closing the gap, significant strain on tissue when it is advanced down to a bone through, postoperative adhesions, infection, deltoid retraction or detachment, denervation of the rotator cuff muscles or deltoid, limited results compared to the patient's expectation, sterile drainage in spite of adequate decompression, concurrent cervical radiculopathy, or syringomyelia.

PROGNOSIS

Most young athletes who have not developed thickening or fibrosis of the cuff, bony spurs under acromion, or significant erosion of the rotator cuff do well in therapy consisting of relative diminishing their activity level, non-steroidal anti-inflammatory medication, mobilization and strengthening within 6 to 8 weeks. It is important to emphasize to these young athletes that they need to continue these stretching and strengthening exercises at home, before and after sport activity so that the pain does not return. It is important to correct the improper mechanics that caused the problem, such as insufficient body roll in swimming or throwing too hard without proper strengthening of the internal and external rotators, scapular stabilizers in pitching, so that symptoms do not redevelop.

If conservative management is not effective, arthroscopic intervention can be done for subacromial decompression, and therapy modified accordingly. That is, if anterior subluxation signs are found, internal rotation strengthening is done first, working toward external rotation strengthening and then elevation strengthening. Even with primary impingement, debridement of the acromion must not be so aggressive as to allow initiation of laxity of the joint where the postoperative response is more variable. Returning to sport activity may take from 2 days to 9 months even after arthroscopic subacromial decompression.

Open procedures that encompass A/C joint surgery and rotator cuff repair will take longer to recover from if the deltoid is taken down in exposure. Deltoid function is important in rehabilitation; and the muscle must heal before attempting strengthening exercises. Obviously, less wear from the A/C joint into the tendon means less injury and an overall better result. If there has been significant wear of the cuff, it is often useful to retrieve the eroded edges and bring them together, in effect thickening the cuff so that it is better balanced and rides more smoothly under the acromion and the muscles work more normally due to centralization of the humeral head.

When treating associated impingement, one is tempted to take down the fibrous area of the non-fused symptomatic acromial apophysis to develop bleeding edges of bone for the healing response. This does not work out well if percutaneous pins and screws are all that is used for acromial fixation, because there is significant motion across the front of the acromion in the activities of daily living.

Associated degenerative arthritis of the acromioclavicular joint must be dealt with effectively and concurrently; otherwise, the mobilization and strengthening necessary to overcome impingement cannot proceed or at least is must less predictable. Continued mobilization and strength to minimize recurrence of symptoms is important, especially to elite athletes.

In the advanced disease state, subacromial decompression or rotator cuff debridement or repair almost universally decrease pain. Subsequent mobility return to athletic activity are directly related to the integrity of the tissue and of the repair and to the amount of motion possible post-surgically. The larger the tear and the poorer the tissue at the time of repair, the less successful the return to athletic activity.

Patient Education

It is important to continue strengthening and stretching to help prevent them from recurring. The athlete who has undergone surgical intervention for symptoms must also be warned that he or she needs to maintain strength and mobility on a lifetime basis to help avoid recurrence of symptoms. The main cause of patients returning to the clinic after successful management of an impingement problem is noncompliance with a home exercise program.

PREVENTION

Many progressive rotator cuff injuries are preventable and that stretching the joint capsule and humeral head depressors and scapular stabilization by medial scapular muscle strengthening and stabilization exercise can diminish or prevent the initiation of impingement symptoms. Proper body mechanics in athletic endeavors is also mandatory. Icing the shoulder before and after activity, stretching, weight training, and weighted pendulum or Codman exercises are also needed. Horizontal flexion and hyperabduction stretching, internal and external rotation strengthening, and functional abduction strengthening are useful to help avoid impingement symptoms.

BIBLIOGRAPHY

1. A modified internal rotation stretching technique for Hover hand and throwing athletes. Johan Sen RL, Callis M. J Orthop Sports Physical Therapy. 1995;21(4):216-9.
2. A narrative review on classification of pain conditions of the upper extremities. Jesper Norregaard, Scndinavion Journal Rehab Medicine, 1998;31:153-64.
3. A self-administered questionnaire for assessment of symptoms and function of the shoulder - John C - Finsalata. Journal of Bone and Joint Surgery. 1997;79A(8).

4. Althechek D, Warren R. Arthoroscopic acromion plasty. J Bone Joint Surgery, 1990;72(A):1198-1207.
5. An electromyographical analysis of the scapular stabilizing synergists during a push up progression - Lear LJ, Gross MT, Jorthop. Sports Physiotherpay 1998;28(3):146-57.
6. An EMG analysis of the shoulder in throwing and pitching a preliminary report. Jobe FW Tibenej, E Perry, Am J Sport Med, 1983;11;3-5.
7. Anatomic relationship in the shoulder impingement syndrome. Clin Orthop, 1993;294:96-102.
8. Arroyo JS, Hershon SJ. Special consideration in the athletic throwing shoulder. Orthop Clin, North Am, 1997;28(1):69-78.
9. Arthur M, Pappas, Richard M, Wawaki and Claire F. Rehabilitation of pitching shoulder, Mccarthy. The American orthopaedics society for sports medicine.
10. Bak K. Non-traumatic glenohumeral instability and coracoacromial impingement in swimmers. Med Sci Sports. 1996;6(3):132-44.
11. Barnes DA, Tullus Hs. An analysis of 100 symptomatic baseball players. Am J Sports Med, 1978;6:63-7.
12. Basmajian JV. Therapeutic exercise. Molone T, Mcpoil T, Nitz A.
13. Beattic PF. Orthopaedic and sports physical therapy. Williams & Wilkins. Mosby Publication. 1978.
14. Biomechanical bash of human movement. Joseph Hamil.
15. Biomechanics of the shoulder joint. Arch. Surg, 1973;107:425-31.
16. Biomechanics of the shoulder, Denies L Hart.
17. Brox JI. Muscle activation after supervised exercises in patients with rotator tendinosis, Arch Phys. Med Rehabil, 2000; 81(1):67-72.
18. Brox JI. Staff, Arthroscopic surgery compared with supervised exercises in patients with rotator cuff disease (stage II impingement syndrome). Br Med J 307:899.
19. Burk DLJ. Karasick, Rotatocuff tears, aprography somegraphy and surgery Am J Roentgenol, 1989;153:86.
20. Burns TP, Turba JE. Arthroscopic Treatment of shoulder impingement in athletes. Am J Sports Med, 1992;20:13-16.
21. Clancy WG Jr (ed): Shoulder problems in overhead overuse sports: Am J. Sports Med. 1979;7:138-44.
22. Clinical kinesiology by brunn storms, 5th Edition, Laurak Smith.
23. Codman EA. The shoulder: rupture of the supraspinatus tendon and other lesions in or about the subacromical bursa. Boston: Thomas Todd. 1934.

24. Collins HR, Lund D. Baseball injuries. In: Schneider RC, Kennedy JC, Plant MC (eds). Sports injuries: Mechanisms, Prevention and treatment. Baltimore; Williams and Wilkins, 1986:64-77.
25. Cook EE, Gray VL, Savinar-Noque E, Medeiros J. Shoulder antagonistic strengthen ratio: A comparison between college level baseball pitchers and nonpitchers. J Orthop Sports Phy Ther. 1987;8(9):451-61.
26. Corso Q. Impingement relief test; an adjunctive procedure to traditional assessment of shoulder impingement syndrome. J Orhop Sports Physther. 1995;22(5)183-92.
27. Cronic rotator cuff impingement in the throwing athlete. Am J Sports Med, 1976;6:231-40.
28. CSII, Flatow EL, Lech O. Tears of the rotator cuff: long term results of anterior acromion plasty and repair: Paper presented at the American shoulder and elbow - Surgeons Fourth Meeting, Atlanta, 1988.
29. Daniels L. Worthinghan's Muscle testing: Techniques of Manual Examination. WB Saunders 2007.
30. Dynamic analysis of throwing shoulders and glenohumeral in stabilities, Ronald Glous man. J Bone and Joint Surgery, 1988;70A:220-5.
31. Frank W Jobe. Serious rotator cuff injuries, symposium on injuries to the shoulder in the athlete clinics of sports medicine, 1983;2(2).
32. Freddic H, David AS. Sports injuries, mechanisms, prevention and treatment 2nd edn. 2001.
33. Freedman L, Munro RR: abduction of the arm in scapular plane: Scapular and glenohumeral movements. J Bone Joint Surgery, 1966;48A:1503-10.
34. Freedom J. Abduction of the arm in the scapular plane scapular and gelno humeral movements. Bone Joint surg, 48A:1503-10.
35. FU FH, Harner CD, Klien AH. Shoulder/impingement syndrome. A critical review. Clin Orthop, 1991;169:162-73.
36. Gainor BT, Pitrowski. The throw: Biomechanics and acute injury Am J Sports Med, 1980;8:114-9.
37. Gainor BT. Piotrowski G, Puhl J, Allen WC, Hagen R. The Throw: Biomechanisms and acute injury. AM J Sports Med, 1987;15:586-90.
38. Hawlains RJ and Kennedy JC. Impingement syndrome in athletes. Am J. Sports Medicine, 1980;8:87.
39. Impingement syndrome in athletic shoulder. Richard J Hokins. Symposium of injuries to the shoulder in athletes, clinics in sports medicine, 1983;2(2).

40. Influence of sports discipline on shoulder rotator cuff balance. Codine P, Bernard PL. Med Sci - Sports exercise, 1997; 29(11):1400-5.
41. Inman VT, Saunders JB, Dec M, Abost LC. Observations on the function of the shoulder joint. Journal of bone joint surgery 1944;26:1-30.
42. Jackson DW. Chronic rotator cuff impingement in the throwing athlete. Orthopaedic Trans 1977;1:24.
43. Jobe FW, Bradley JP. Rotator cuff injuries in baseball; prevention and rehabilitation. Sports Med, 1988;6:377-87.
44. Jobe FW, Moynes DR, Tibone JE, tal. Can EMA analysis of the shoulder in throwing and pitching. A preliminary report. Am J. sports med, 11:3-5.
45. Jobe FW, Radovich Moynes D. Delineation of diagnostic criteria and a rehabilitation program for rotator cuff injuries. Am J Sports Med, 1982;10:336-9.
46. Jobe FW, Tibone JE, Jobe CM, K Vitne RS. The shoulder in sports. In: Rockwood CA; Matsen FA (eds). The shoulder. Philadelphia: WB Saunders, 1990;961-90.
47. Jobe FW, Yucum LA, Moynes DR, et al. Shoulder and arm exercises for baseball players. Biomechanics laboratory, sentinel hospital medical centre, Inglewood, CA, 1983.
48. Joint structure and function - A comprehensive analysis, Norkins.
49. Kronberg M, Nemeth G, Broström LA. Muscle activity and coordination in the shoulder. (An Electromyographic study) Margareta Kronberg, Gunnar Nemeth. Clin Orthop Relat Res. 1990;257:76-85.
50. Kulund DN, MC Cue FW. Tennis injuries: Prevention and treatment Am J Sports Med, 1999;7:249-53.
51. Lipsomb AB. Baseball pitching injuries in growing athletes. Am J Sports Med, 1975;3:25-34.
52. Lipsomb AB. Baseball pitching injuries in growing athletes. Am J Sports Med, 1975;3:25-34.
53. Lukasiewicz AC, Mcclurep, Jorthop. Comparison of 3 - dimensional scapular and orientation between subjects with or without shoulder impingement. Sports Physiotherapy, 1999;29(10):574-83.
54. Maria Zulmaga O. Sports physiotherapy - Applied Science and Practice. Churchill & Livingstone 1995.
55. Masala S, Fanucci E, Maiotti M, Nardocci M, et al. Impingement syndrome of the shoulder - Clinical data and radiologic fundings. Radiol Med. 1995;89(1-2):18-21.
56. Meister K. Injuries to the shoulder in the throwing athlete part one - Biomechanics, Pathophysiology and classification of injury. Am J Sports Med, 2000;28(2):265-75.

57. Morrison DS. Non-operative treatment of subacromial impingement syndrome. J Bone Joint surg Am. 1997;79(5):732-7.
58. Muscular imbalance and shoulder pain in volleyball attackers. Kugler A Reinigers British Journal of sports Med, 1996;30(3):256-9.
59. Near CS. Anterior acromioplasty for chronic impingement syndrome in the shoulder J. Bone Joint Surgery, 1972;54A:41.
60. Neer CS II. Anterior acropmioplasty for the chronic impingement syndrome in the shoulder. A preliminary report. J Bone Joint, 1972;54A:41-50.
61. Neer CSII, Flatow, Lech O. Tears of the rotator cuff: long term results of anterior acrominoplasty and repair: Paper presented at American shoulder and elbow - surgeons 4th meeting, Atlanta, 1988.
62. Nirschi RP. Rotator cuff tendonitis: Basic concepts of pathoetiology (American Academy of orthopedic surgerious instructional course Lecture No. 439. Las Vegas, W: 1989;4405.
63. Noah J, Gudumal R; Rotator cuff injuries in the throwing athlete Orhtop Review. 1988;17:1091-6.
64. O' Donogue DH. Treatment of injuries to athletes. Philadelphia: WB Saunders, 1984;433-46.
65. O' Donogue DH. Treatment of injuries to athletes. Philadelphia: WB Saunders, 1984;433-46.
66. Pappas AM, Zawaski RM, MC Carthy CF. Rehabilitation of the pitching shoulder. Am J Sports Med, 1985;13:223-35.
67. Pappas Am. Biomechanics of baseball pitching. Am. Journal of Sports Medicine, 1985;13:216-22.
68. Patterns of flexibility, laxity and strength in Normal shoulders and shoulders with instability and impingement. Am J Sports Med, 1990;18:366-75.
69. Poppen NK, Walker PS. Normal and Abnormal motion of the shoulder. J Bone Joint Surgery (AM), 1976;58:195.
70. Prevention of injury to the shoulder through exercises and therapy; - Diane Radovich Moyuos; symposium on injuries to the shoulder in the athletes. Clinics in sports medicine: 1983;2(2).
71. Priest JD, Nagal. Tennis shoulder. Am J Sports Med. 1976;4:28-42.
72. Rahme H, Solem - Bertoft E, Scand J. The subacromial impingement syndrome - Rihabil Med, 1998;30(4):253-62.
73. Rathbur JB, MC Nab I. The microvascular pattern of the rotator cuff. J Bone Joint Surgery, 1970;32B:540-53.
74. Recruitment patterns of the scapular rotator muscles in freestyle swimmers with subacromial impingement - Wadsworth DJ, Bullock - Saxton JE, Int J sports Med, 1997;18(8):618-24.
75. Richard J, Hawkins E, Hobeika. Impingement syndrome in athletic shoulder clinics of Sp. Med, 1983;2(2).

76. Richard KN RYV, Cormick MC. An EMG analysis of shoulder function in tennis players. Am Journal of Sp. Med, 1988;16(5).
77. Richard KN, Mc Cornick J, Jobe FW, Movens DR, Antonelli DJ. An electromyographic analysis of shoulder function in tennis players. The American Journal of Sports Medicine. 1988;16(5):481-5.
78. Rodin E. Relevant Biomechanics in the treatment of musculo-skeletal injuries and disorder. Clin Orthopaedics, 1980;146:2.
79. Role of scapular stabilizers in etiology and treatment of impingement syndrome schmilt IL, Snyder - Mckler L. J Orthop Sports Phys. Ther 1999;29(1):31-8.
80. Rotator cuff injuries in baseball; prevention and rehabilitation: Jobe FW, Bradley Sports Med, 1988;6:3777-389.
81. Rotator cuff pathology in athletes - Blevius FT. Sports Med 1997; 24(3):205-20.
82. Saha AK: Mechanism of shoulder movements and a plea for the recognition of "Zero position" of the glenohumeral joint. Clin Orthop, 1983;173:3-10.
83. Sain J, Andrews JR. Proper pitching techniques. In: Zarins B, Andrews Jr, Carson WG (eds). Injuries to throwing arm. Philadelphia: WB Saunders, 1985;31-7.
84. Samilson RL, Binder WF. Symptomatic full thickness. Tears of the rotator cuff: an analysis 292 shoulders in 276 patients. Orthopaedic Clin North Am, 1975;6:449-66.
85. Shoulder impingement syndromes in athletes and their surgical management. Am J Sports Med, 1981;9:11-5.
86. Shoulder rehabilitation - Equipment modification. J of Sp. Physical Therapy, 1985.
87. Shrode LW. Treating shoulder impingement using the supraspinatus synchronization exercise. J Manipulative Physio Ther, 1994;17(1):43-53.
88. Stephen M, Howell, Brian J, Galinat J. Normal and abnormal mechanics of glenohumeral joint in horizontal plane. Bone joint surgery (A), 1988.
89. The painful shoulder semin. Arthritis Rheum, 1977;7:21-47.
90. Tibone JE, Elrood B, Jobe FW, et al. Surgical treatment of rotator cuff in athletes. J Bone and Joint Surgery, 1986;68a:887-91
91. Tibone JE, Elrood B, Jobe FW, et al. surgical treatment of the rotator cuff in Athletes. J Bone Joint Surgery, 1986;68A:887-91.
92. Ticker JB. Recognition and treatment of refractory. Posterior capsular contracture of the shoulder. Arthroscopy, 2000;16(1):27-34.
93. Tullos HS and King JW. Throwing mechanism in sports. Orthop. Clin North America, 1973;3:709-30.

94. Turkel SJ, Panio NW, Mrshall JL, Guergis FG. Stabilizing mechanics preventing anterior dislocation of the glenohumeral Jt. J Bone Joint Surgery. 1981;63:1208-17.
95. Turkels J, Panio J. Stabilizing Mechanisms preventing anterior dislocation of the glenohumeral joint. Bone and Joint Surgery, 1981;63:1208-17.
96. Uhtoff HK, Loehr J, Sarkar K. The pathogenesis of rotator cuff tears. In: Taka Gishi N Cd. The shoulder. Tokyo: Tokyo professional postgraduate services, 1987;211.

Chapter

10

Brachial Plexus Injury

Brachial plexus is attached by fascia to the first rib medially and to the coracoid process laterally, so that side flexion of the head with shoulder depression stretches the upper plexus (C5-C6) and compresses it against the first rib, known as Erb's palsy. It commonly occurs during the last phase of vaginal delivery, in case of narrow maternal pelvis and/or disproportionately large fetal shoulders. Pulling the head to facilitate the delivery results in excessive widening of the angle between neck and shoulder. Incidence of obstetrical brachial plexus injury is 1 per 1000 birth - in poor medical facility. The forces seem to act with diminishing violence from C5 downwards to T1. The lesions are always supraclavicular and not associated with vascular damage as in adult. Lesions to the phrenic nerve, accessory nerve, rupture of scalene or sternocleido-mastoid muscles and fracture of clavicle and humerus may uncommonly be associated with obstetrical brachial plexus injury. Brain and spinal cord injuries are uncommon. It occurs in adults due to fall on the shoulder tip from high velocity motor bike accident, which results in excessive separation of the neck and shoulder. C5-C6 lesion results in paralysis of rhomboids, levator scapulae, serratus anterior, supraspinatus, infraspinatus, deltoid, biceps brachii, brachioradialis and supinator. The attitude of the limb is shoulder adduction, internal rotation, elbow straight, and forearm pronation, typical policeman's tip/waiter's tip position (Fig. 10.1). Functional deficit includes inability to abduct the

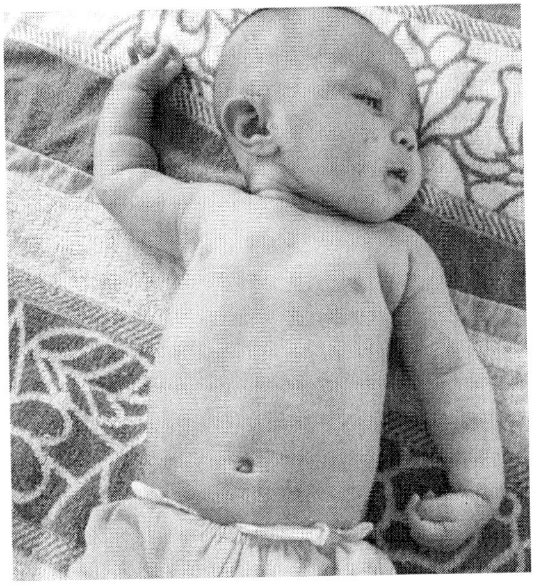

Fig. 10.1: Attitude of limb in a typical obstetrical brachial plexus injury

shoulder, flex and supinate the elbow. Wrist extension may or may not be involved.

BRACHIAL PLEXUS

Roots: Anterior primary rami of C5, C6, C7, C8 and T1 spinal nerve roots form the brachial plexus. Dorsal scapular nerve (C5) supplying the rhomboids (scapular retraction) and long thoracic nerve (C5, C6 and C7 mainly C5) to serratus anterior (protraction of scapula) originate from the root level (Fig. 10.2).

Trunks: The roots form the trunks. C5 and C6 nerve roots join to form the upper trunk, C7 continues as middle trunk and C8 and T1 roots form the lower trunk. Suprascapular nerve (C5) originates from the upper trunk and supplies supraspinatus (shoulder abduction) and infraspinatus (external rotation). Nerve to subclavius (C5 and C6) also originates from upper trunk (Fig. 10.2).

Divisions and Cords: Each trunk is divided into anterior and posterior divisions. Anterior divisions of upper and middle trunks combine to form the lateral cord, anterior division of

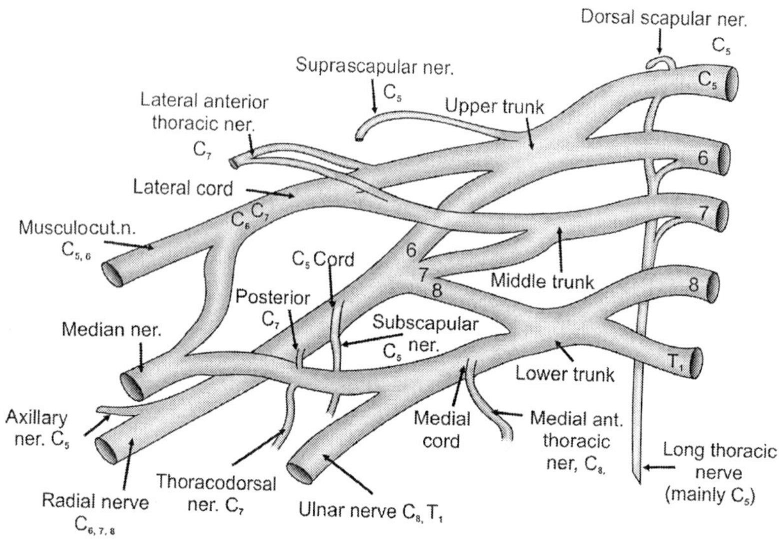

Fig. 10.2: Brachial plexus

lower trunk form the medial cord and posterior divisions of all the trunks unite to form the posterior cord. Lateral pectoral nerve (C5, C6 and C7) supplying pectorals and musculocutaneous nerve (C5, C6 and C7) supplying coracobrachialis, biceps brachi and brachialis originate from the lateral cord. Medial pectoral nerve (C8 and T1), medial cutaneous nerve of arm (C8 and T1), medial cutaneous nerve of forearm (C8 and T1), ulnar nerve (C7, C8 and T1) originate from the medial cord. Lateral root of median (C5, C6 and C7) originating from the lateral cord and medial root of median (C8 and T1) originating from the lateral cord combine to form the median nerve. Upper subscapular and lower subscapular nerves (C5, C6) supplying subscapularis and teres major, thoracodorsal nerve (C6, C7 and C8) supplying latissimus dorsi, axillary nerve (C5, C6) supplying deltoid and teres minor, radial nerve (C5, C6, C7, C8 and T1) arise from the posterior cord (Fig. 10.2).

Excessive hyperabduction stretches the lower plexus (C7-T1), known as Klumpke's palsy. Many babies in breech presentation may develop obstetrical brachial plexus injury apparently caused by forceful pulling of the upper limb to facilitate the delivery. In adults, it may occur due to fall on outstretched hand, hanging by grasping some overhead object. There develops paralysis of intrinsic muscles of hand due to involvement of combined median nerve and ulnar nerve. A claw hand deformity develops by the unopposed pull of long finger flexors in the absence of intrinsics. Functional deficit includes inability to flex and extend the fingers.

Secondarily, there develops atrophy of the paralyzed muscles, overstretching of the paralyzed muscles with loss of their elasticity, adoptive shortening of the intact muscles with loss of their extensibility, bony deformities, etc. complications. Severity of injury varies from mild stretching with edema or hemorrhage with scar blocking the nerve impulses (neuropraxia) to axonal rupture (axonotmesis) or avulsion of nerve root from the spinal cord. Stretching of axons without rupture recovers spontaneously as the edema subsides. In case of axonal separation there is Wallerian degeneration followed by regeneration at the rate of 1 mm per day, but unlikely to recover completely regardless of level of injury. Usually the prognosis of Erb's palsy is best of all types of brachial plexus injury. Usually, it recovers within 4–5 months. If no deltoid or biceps recovery has occurred by 3rd months, the prognosis is poor. In case of Klumpke's palsy full recovery is unlikely. A whole plexus injury has an extremely poor prognosis for recovery. In root avulsion, spontaneous recovery does not take place.

CLASSIFICATION

Obstetrical brachial plexus injury may be partial, i.e upper trunk palsy or a more or less complete paralysis of the whole limb. This is not really relevant for the future course though the more extensive the palsy the more probable it is that the upper trunk has been severely affected. Classification is done 2–3 weeks after birth. The classification assesses the future of the palsy and will exclude many mild cases which recover full function in a matter of days.

Group I

The newborn presents with a typical Erb's palsy with paralysis of abductor and external rotators, flexors of the elbow and supinators of forearm, frequently a part of wrist extensors. There is no Horner's sign and the fingers and wrist have normal flexors, the intrinsic muscles of the hand are not affected.

Usually in this group the newborn will start to recover function before the end of first month. At 4–6 months the infant presents a normal extremity. Sunderland I, III and exceptionally 3 to the upper trunk is probable in these lesions.

Group II

There is same picture as group I but active elbow extension is not as strong since C7 is partially affected. There is no sign of recovery in shoulder and elbow flexion before the 1st month. From then the infant will recover steadily but may develop a contracture in internal rotation and adduction at the shoulder requiring surgery at 6–8 months. Sunderland II, III to upper trunk and degree I and II to the C7 root.

If well treated, these children will have minor sequelae later but the humerus is always 2–3cm shortened by the age of 6 years. Differential diagnosis between I and II are made at 6 weeks of age, the former is recovered but the latter is not.

Group III

In this group, palsy affects almost whole limb at birth and at 1 month the infant has a flail shoulder with internal rotation of the humerus. No elbow flexion and weak extension. The wrist is flexed and fist closely tight. There is no Horner's sign. The hand will improve slowly and finally to gain good function. Recovery at the shoulder will be slow, the deltoid remaining paralyzed sometimes for a few years and often remaining functionally poor afterwards while the external rotator nerve recover or may take 14–15 months to have any significant function. If not treated properly these infants stiffen their shoulder only using scapulothoracic movement to full extent.

These babies have rupture or severe stretch injury in continuity of the upper trunk. III and sometimes IV degree injury to C7 and C8 occur and T1 is less affected. Only about 15% will recover satisfactory function. Shoulder movement will be limited and require palliative surgery. A 30° flexion deformity of the elbow is common and growth of scapula and humerus will be limited by about 10%.

Group IV

This group was previously divided into two groups one without Horner's sign, the other with Horner's sign; but it has been found that there are no significant differences between them regarding the late sequelae.

At birth, there is complete paralysis of C5–T1 and the infant will present a flail extremity up to 6–8 months (little finger movement). Later at around 1 year some finger function may reappear either because T1 was not avulsed or because there is an important anastomosis T2.

Surgical exploration has shown a wide variety of severe lesions. There is always a rupture of C5, a rupture or infrequency avulsion of C6. Usually C7–C8 are completely avulsed and T1 incompletely. Various combinations of ruptures or avulsions are possible and explain the poor pattern of recovery. Growth of the arm will be retarded 6–8 cm by adolescence.

SUNDERLAND CLASSIFICATION

First Degree (Class I)

It is a temporary interruption of conduction without loss of axon continuity. There is sensory motor problems distal to the site of injury. Recovery occurs completely within days to weeks. EMG shows lack of fibrillation potential and positive sharpwaves.

Second Degree (Class II)

Class II involves loss of relative continuity of the axon and its covering of myelin, but preservation of epineurium and perineurium. Wallerian degeneration occurs distal to the site of injury. Here is sensory motor deficit, no nerve conduction distal to the site of injury 3-4 days after injury. EMG shows fibrillation potentials and positive sharp waves. 2-3 weeks after injury, axonal regeneration occurs. Sometimes surgical intervention is required because of scar tissues.

Third Degree (Class II)

It is a nerve fibre interruption. Here is lesion of the endoneurium, but the epineurium and perineurium intact. Recovery is possible, but surgical intervention may be required.

Fourth Degree (Class II)

Only epineurium remain intact and requires surgery.

Fifth Degree (Class III)

It is a complete transection of the nerve and requires surgery.

HORNER'S SYNDROME

Horner's syndrome is the combination of ptosis, constriction of pupil (miosis), sometimes accompanied by anhydrosis of the face, flushing of the face on the affected side. It is due to deficiency of sympathetic activity suggestive of pregangtionic lesion.

EVALUATION

A thorough systemic evaluation is essential to assess accurately the nature and extent of brachial plexus lesion and to develop an appropriate and effective treatment plan.

History

Detailed history regarding occupation, handedness, mode of onset, duration, mechanism of injury and history of pain including the site, nature, intensity by visual analogue scale. Period of loss of consciousness at the time of injury, associated injury such as fracture, vascular injury, head injury, etc. has to be taken.

Physical Evaluation

Detail neuromuscular evaluation include posture, attitude of the limb/deformity, passive joint range of motion, tightness/ contracture, active range of motion, muscle strength by manual muscle testing, sensation, coordination, activities of daily living, disability, edema, peripheral pulsations, Tinel's sign, etc.

Tinel's sign demonstrated by tapping from distal to proximal along the course of the nerve and note the tingling sensation experienced by the patient. A distal Tinel's sign indicates a lesion in continuity, where the axonal connections within the nerve trunk are intact. Presence of strong localized tenderness above the clavicle indicates a possible neuroma resulting from disruption of part of the plexus, where the prognosis is poor.

Investigations

Lumbar puncture - Xanthochromic CSF indicates root avulsions.

Myelography and magnetic resonance imaging is used to indicate the status of the nerve roots in the presence of traction injuries to the brachial plexus, i.e. to exclude root avulsion.

X-ray may show, increase distance between acromion and humeral metaphysis, retardation of growth, deformity of shoulder joint, dislocation of radial head.

Electrodiagnostic investigations such as needle electromyography, nerve conduction velocity, Faradic - galvanic test, and strength duration curve are useful.

Needle electromyography of the paraspinal muscles is appropriate in determining root avulsion. Posterior cervical musculature is serially innervated by the posterior primary rami of the same level spinal nerves innervating the anterior primary rami that make up the plexus. Therefore denervated limb musculature but innervated erector spinae muscles corresponding to that level indicates posterior primary rami of the same level is intact. It confirms postganglionic lesion. Denervation of both limb musculature and erector spinae indicates preganglionic lesion. Absence of fibrillation activity several weeks after nerve injury is suggestive of good prognosis.

EMG at 3–4 weeks confirm neuropraxia showing residual motor unit indicating good prognosis, at 2 months shows possible signs of re-innervation. Recording of evoked sensory potential is useful to ascertain root avulsion. Preserved sensory conduction due to intact dorsal root ganglion in the absence of motor conduction in NCV study indicates root avulsion.

F-G test and S-D curve allows the clinician to assess neuromuscular recovery.

Preganglionic root avulsion is characterized by high speed impact injury, a period of loss of consciousness, positive Horner's sign, presence of sensory action potential, presence of meningoceles on myelogram, pain on the anesthetic part, associated vascular, bony and head injuries. Whereas postganglionic nerve lesion is characterized by low speed impact injury, no loss of consciousness, negative Horner's sign, absence of sensory action potential, normal myelogram, no pain and no associated injury. Pain in preganglionic nerve root lesion usually develops 2–3 weeks after injury characterized by constant burning or crushing type of pain over the involved dermatome. Sometimes suddenly severe pain develops, which lasts. Patient finds difficulty to sleep, but once asleep, does not awakened by pain.

Conservative Treatment

Aim of management includes prevention of soft tissues contracture, shoulder subluxation, injury to insensitive part, etc. secondary complications.

Initially the extremity must be supported to prevent shoulder subluxation. No passive range of motion exercises is to be given for several days to allow the traumatic neuritis to resolve. Additional trauma and further injury can be prevented by avoiding abduction and posterior projection of the shoulder and the limb must be supported when holding the baby. The extremity is either left along the side of the newborn when supine or put across the chest with elbow flexed in a sleeve or jersey, while the other joints are frequently mobilized. The shoulder is put at rest for 3 weeks. Contractures are not likely to occur in such a short time. Then passive range of motion exercises in various planes are given gently to prevent adoptive shortening. Normal biomechanics, i.e. normal glenohumeral rhythm after about 30 degrees of abduction, humeral external rotation at about 60 degrees of abduction has to be followed to prevent damage to the shoulder. Parents are taught to move the joints gently and particularly to widen the humeroscapular

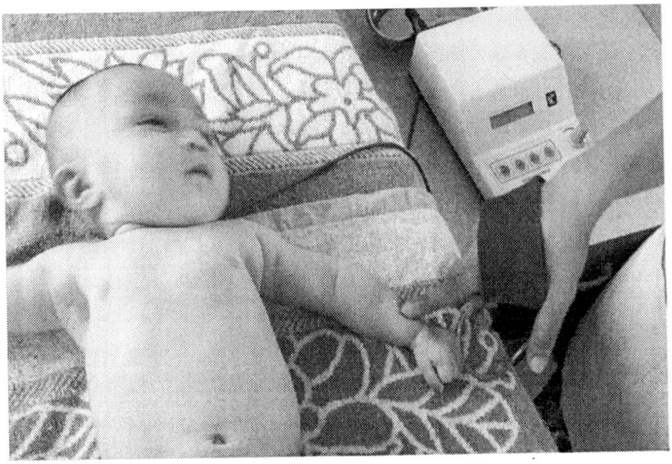

Fig. 10.3: Electrical stimulation

angle. It is good that they touch the affected limb to provide sensory feedback, which is very important.

Use of splint is controversial in Erb's palsy. The affected extremity is usually splinted with the arm abducted to 90 degrees externally rotated and elbowflexed to 90 degrees by stitching/buttoning velcro straps to the bed sheet. But there is risk of injury to the shoulder due to movements.

Electrotherapy is controversial, efficient electrical stimulation is badly tolerated. Interrupted galvanic stimulation to the paralytic muscles may be given to maintain their physiological properties, prevent fibrosis and atrophy. The active electrode is placed over the dorsum of the therapist's hand and electrical stimulation is applied by the therapist's finger, so that the intensity of the current can be controlled well. Passive electrode is placed on the baby's body (Fig. 10.3).

Pain due to preganglionic lesion often gets relieved with time. It can be managed by TENS. The active electrode is placed either over the appropriate damaged dermatome or more distally in case that area is an anesthetic.

Active movements of the uninvolved movements must be encouraged. As the nerve recovers and the paralytic muscles start contracting, movements in gravity eliminated plane progressed to antigravity movement and then resisted movements are given. Then functional activities are incorporated.

Operative Treatment

Surgical repair of plexus (microsurgery) is indicated in group III and IV, if biceps fail to show sign of recovery between 3 and 4 months or in a completely flail arm with horner's syndrome after 1 month. Following nerve grafting, the limb is immobilized across the chest in a soft dressing for 3 weeks.

In adults with brachial plexus injury surgery is indicated only when there is no sign of recovery clinically or from electromyography within first 6 months of injury. Microsurgery using autograft, usually sural nerve occasionally medial cutaneous nerve of forearm, is considered. Recovery of elbow flexion between 1 year to 11/2 years of surgery is considered successful. Most patients will not be able to raise their arms overhead following surgery. Lower plexus repair is rarely performed because by the time nerve growth is complete fibrosis of the intrinsic muscles of hand will occur.

Palliative surgery during conservative treatment usually first considered around the age of 5 months. If the passive movement shows a steady decrease of maximal humero-scapular angle, a contracture of subscapularis and possibly teres major is developing. When no improvement is obtained by intensifying exercises and passive mobilization, a release of subscapularis from the scapula and possibly a lengthening of teres major and contracted facial bands in the axilla is indicated until full passive range of motion is obtained. The operation is done through a posterior axillary incision and the scar is acceptable even for girls. The operation is performed even when the infant is one year old. Immobilization in external rotation is maintained for at least 3 weeks adding 1 week for every 2 months of age above 6 months, i.e. 4 weeks for a child of 8 months, 6 weeks for a child of 10 months, and 6 weeks for 1 year child. Anterior and posterior dislocation of the humeral head will not occur if this is done. Results will be less convincing in children older than this. After immobilization PT should be continued until the age of 2 years.

The second palliative surgery during conservative treatment may be considered between 18 and 24 months when good shoulder movement has not been obtained and enough active muscles are available to consider transfer. Very careful pre-operative evaluation is necessary for success. The key muscle is deltoid. If its function is poor or nil and that of supraspinatus is good, only limited movements are obtained whatever the transfer. The latissimus dorsi if functional, can substitute for the posterior deltoid but requires an extensive exposure. The humeral tendon of the latissimus dorsi is attached near to the insertion of deltoid and spine of scapula while the teres major is transferred to the minor. An alternative is shoulder arthrodesis, one can manage to do functional activities by compensatory scapular movements using trapezius, serratus anterior. Humeral derotational osteotomy is considered to correct shoulder internal rotation or forearm pronation deformity to improve the functional activities.

If the deltoid function is good but that of supraspinatus is poor, transfer of the upper trapezius into the later and of the latissimus dorsi and teres major into the infraspinatus and teres minor may improve function dramatically. Such surgery may not be possible in children with group III and IV plexus injury.

For elbow flexion, Clarks transfer should be done for female babies (pectoralis major to biceps). Zancolli's technique - latissimus dorsi to biceps may be considered. Steindler's should be avoided.

BIBLIOGRAPHY

1. Donatelli RA: Physical therapy of the shoulder, 2nd edition; Churchill Livingstone, 1991.
2. Joshi and Kotwal: Essentials of orthopaedics and Applied Physiotherapy, 1st edition; BI Churchill Livingstone Pvt. Ltd, 1999.
3. Saidofff DC: Critical pathways in therapeutic intervention. Mosby, 2002.

Chapter

11

Physiotherapy in Surgical Conditions

TOTAL SHOULDER ARTHROPLASTY

Arthroplasty is surgical reconstruction of a painless, movable, stable and functional joint. In 1826, John Rhea Barton was the first to perform osteotomy of the hip to allow movements and promote functional pseudoarthrosis in a malpositioned stiff hip. It was the first true joint arthroplasty. In 1867, Louis Xavier Edouard Leopold Ollier performed functional pseudoarthrosis by the interposition of soft tissue at an osteotomy site. Then Murphy reported 84 arthroplasties of various joints with the insertion of local flaps of fascia and fatty tissue. William Baer performed arthroplasty extensively by using free fascial flaps composed of chromicised pig bladder, a foreign but absorbable material similar to chromic suture. The advantages of Baer's method over Murphy are that it could be performed through smaller incision and was less difficult. McAusland described a technique for shoulder arthroplasty by using free flap to form a painless, stable and movable, functional joint. Interposition/excision arthroplasty persisted as the standard into early 1930s.

The first total shoulder replacement arthroplasty was performed in 1893 by Jules Pean following report in 1890 by Themistockles Gluck of using custom ivory hemiarthroplasties for reconstruction of knee, elbow and wrist joints. Marius Nygaard Smith-Peterson in 1923 used Vitallium in the development of the cup or mould for hip arthroplasty, which remained the treatment of choice for hip arthritis for the next 30 years. It led to the development of shoulder arthroplasty by E Jonsson and later by Varian. From the late 1930s through late 1950s, a number of appliances were developed for the treatment not only of degenerative arthritis of hip but also fractures. In 1951, Krueger reported use of an anatomically designed humeral head for the treatment of osteonecrosis. In 1952, Richard and associates reported use of acrylic appliances to replace the proximal humerus in a case of fracture-dislocation of humerus. In 1953, deAnquin, Argentina, also inserted an acrylic appliance. In 1955, Charles S Neer reported use of endoprosthesis in the treatment of fracture-dislocation and post-traumatic arthritis. John Charnley reported use of low friction total hip replacement through the use of a high density polyethylene liner fixed with acrylic cement and taking steps to lower the infection rate. Charnley's work had enormous impact on all major joint reconstructions.

Total shoulder prosthesis are classified into three types: Constrained, semiconstrained, and unconstrained. Constrained total shoulder prosthesis is designed with an inherently stable fulcrum, i.e. humeral and glenoid components are linked together, where deltoid elevates the arm without the assistance from the rotator cuff. It is indicated only when rotator cuff mechanism is insufficient or cannot be repaired. Lack of rolling, gliding and rotation transmits the torsional force to the bone-prosthesis interface leading to loosening. Now it is rarely indicated because of high incidence of complications and limited success.

The first unconstrained shoulder prosthesis, the Neer II, was introduced in 1973. Unconstrained implies resurfacing of the articular surfaces. There is no linkage system between the humeral and glenoid components. It allows normal arthrokinesiology and provides greater freedom of movement. The unconstrained prosthesis is relied on the normal anatomy of the shoulder joint to provide stability. It is indicated only when rotator cuff mechanism is intact or can be repaired to provide stability. Unconstrained replacement may be accompanied by acromionectomy to prevent impingement.

The surgery is performed through an anterior deltopectoral incision extending from AC joint to deltoid insertion. The pectoralis major is released, an anterior capsulotomy is performed, humerus is dislocated and excised. Then humeral stem component is fixed in the humeral canal either by bone cement or press fit for fixation. The glenoid fossa is debrided and the glenoid component is fixed by bone cement or press fit for fixation.

Indications

A variety of conditions affect the shoulder, causing progressive loss of the articular cartilage. The resultant arthritis may be accompanied by other pathologic changes such as bone loss, capsular laxity or contracture and rotator cuff rupture resulting in pain, loss of motion, instability and impairment of function. The mainstay of medical management is non-steroidal anti-inflammatory drugs, nutritional supplementation with glucosamine and chondroitin sulfate, oral steroids or other immunosuppressive medications, intra-articular corticosteroid injections and physiotherapy. Once the conservative management fails, surgical options can be considered. Shoulder synovectomy has been used for the rheumatoid disease before the involvement of articular cartilage, which relieves the pain but not the stiffness. Excision arthroplasty was method of choice for the management of septic arthritis, but it results in instability and poor function. Arthrodesis of gleno-humeral joint was the method of management for arthritic conditions of shoulder prior to resurfacing arthroplasty, but it results in significant functional deficits with the limitation of over head activities and functions requiring rotation. The primary indication of shoulder arthroplasty is pain relief, i.e. patients with disabling pain not responding to medical treatment and secondarily to improve motion and functions. Shoulder replacement arthroplasty is contraindicated in chronic infections of the joint, combined paralysis of deltoid and rotator cuff, uncontrolled instability of the joint and neuropathic joint.

Osteoarthritis: Up to 60% of patients undergoing total shoulder arthroplasty carry a diagnosis of primary osteo-arthritis, which is characterized by progressive degeneration of articular cartilage with narrowing of joint space, capsular fibrosis, marginal osteophyte formation mostly along the inferior and posterior margins of the humeral head, subchondral sclerosis, and erosion of posterior glenoid leading to posterior instability. There may be rotator cuff rupture and contracture of subscapularis.

Rheumatoid Arthritis: Rheumatoid arthritis is the second common diagnosis for patients undergoing total shoulder arthroplasty. RA is characterized by synovitis and pannus formation, and subsequent release of inflammatory mediators resulting in the destruction of bone and soft tissue. There may be rotator cuff rupture.

Traumatic Arthritis: Arthritis secondary to displaced fracture and fracture-dislocation of glenohumeral joint.

Osteonecrosis: Osteonecrosis of the head of humerus results from avascularity due to prolonged corticosteroid use, sickle cell anemia, and alcoholism. It can be idiopathic also.

Rotator Cuff Arthropathy: Rotator cuff arthropathy is characterized by massive rotator cuff tear, glenohumeral arthritis, instability and proximal migration of humeral head.

Postoperative Physiotherapy

Postoperative physiotherapy in case of cemented replacement arthroplasty starts immediately. On the first postoperative day active wrist, hand and elbow exercises should be encouraged. Continuous passive motion can be given for early mobilization. Passive and assisted exercises are given on the first post-operative day. Movements in all planes except internal rotation and extension, and external rotation is limited to the amount determined intraoperatively that will not jeopardize the subscapularis repair. Elevation is done in the plane of scapula. No resisted exercise or passive stretching should be given before 6 weeks to allow subscapularis to heal. Sometimes abduction braces are used for the patients with rotator cuff repair and require to be protected from active motion for about 6 weeks. Patients must be cautioned to avoid using hand for push up while getting up from the bed or from sitting, which requires strong contraction of subscapularis. After 6 weeks patient can initiate internal rotation and gentle resisted exercise. For resisted exercise the elbow should be flexed to start with. Rubber tubing is useful for resisted exercises. Weight and pulley circuit can be used both for mobility as well as strengthening. At 12 weeks, all restrictions are lifted, but patients are cautioned not to participate in contact activities and aggressive weight training. Short term complications such as pain and swelling can be managed by ice and may require modification of exercise program.

In case of non-cemented replacement shoulder is immobilized with the arm by the side internally rotated and slightly flexed and elbow flexed in the sling. If TSR is accompanied by rotator cuff repair, the arm is immobilized in abduction splint or pillow for 3 weeks. During immobilization phase active wrist hand and forearm movements should be initiated immediate postoperatively. After 3 weeks, initiate active-assisted and passive shoulder movements. Open kinetic chain active shoulder movements can be performed after 6 weeks.

Complications

The incidences of postoperative complications of total shoulder arthroplasty are relatively less (10.4%) as compared to other major joint replacements. The most effective means of preventing complications are meticulous preoperative planning, skilled surgeon, proper patient selection, proper postoperative management and patient education.

Fracture

Intraoperative fracture shaft of humerus (0.9%) is the result of torque on the arm producing spiral fracture of the reamed canal, which must be stabilized for successful rehabilitation. Fracture of the glenoid is extremely rare and occurs in osteoporotic bones, e.g. rheumatoid arthritis.

Nerve injury

Axillary nerve is most commonly injured during surgery. Radial nerve may be injured due to intraoperative fracture shaft of humerus. Musculocutaneous nerve may be injured due to prolonged retraction on the conjoint tendon complex. Most of the nerve injuries are neurapraxia and recovers spontaneously. It is suggested to observe for 3--6 weeks, then EMG should be done if there is no recovery. Surgical exploration may be considered, if there is no recovery after 3 months.

Malpositioning of the Components

Placing the total shoulder prosthesis components in less than the anatomical position may lead to decreased range of motion or instability.

Instability

Component instability may occur in any direction and may be of different degrees of subluxation or dislocation (1.5%). Superior migration of the humeral component is a very common postoperative complication. It may occur due to imbalance in the force couple between deltoid and surgically treated rotator cuff. It may give rise to loosening of glenoid component. Anterior instability may be caused by the selection of a smaller than the required humeral head component. It may be associated with torn subscapularis. If the patient can place his hand behind the back and not able to lift it, then the tendon is considered as torn. Posterior instability may be caused by the component malpositioning, i.e. placing the glenoid component in too much retroversion. Inferior instability results from excessive removal of proximal humerus, and it leads to weakness of deltoid and impairment of arm elevation past the horizontal plane.

Infection

Infection complicating shoulder arthroplasty is rare (0.4%). Infection during 3–6 weeks postoperatively should be managed by judicious irrigation, debridement and appropriate antibiotics. Chronic infection requires removal of implant, irrigation, debridement and appropriate antibiotics followed by reimplantation with the use of antibiotics with the cement.

Rotator Cuff Tear

Rotator cuff tear is most common complication following total shoulder arthroplasty (1.9%). Patients with small tear complain of pain and require arthrography for the diagnosis. It should be managed by surgical repair. Large tears will cause superior subluxation and loosening of glenoid component. Repair of large tears may not be possible and managed by a salvage procedure with the removal of glenoid component, bone grafting of the glenoid cavity defect and allowing the humeral prosthesis to migrate superiorly.

Loosening of the Prosthesis

Loosening of glenoid component is more common after total shoulder arthroplasty, which is characterized by radiolucent lines around the bone-cement interface, pain and impairment of function. Loosening of humeral component is characterized by progressive radiolucent line and change in implant position.

Stiffness

Post operative stiffness is rare except if the long-term joint contracture is not corrected preoperatively. It should be managed by physiotherapy. Manipulation is contraindicated as it may cause rotator cuff tear or loosening of prosthesis.

Progressive loss of motion can be managed by capsulectomy and Z-lengthening of subscapularis if required.

Heterotopic Ossification

Heterotopic ossifican is a rare complication, which is characterized by formation of bone at ectopic soft tissue, pain and progressive limitation of range of motion. The cause is not known. Mobilization worsens the condition and it improves with rest. In case of extensive ossification with impairment of function surgery followed by radiation treatment and use of indocin have been reported to be beneficial.

Flailed Shoulder Arthroplasty

Flailed shoulder arthroplasty is difficult to manage and the results of revision arthroplasty are inferior to the primary arthroplasty.

SYNOVECTOMY

Synovectomy may be considered in case of chronic synovitis with persistent pain, not responding to medical management. It should be done before the articular cartilage is involved. Chronic synovitis is characterized by swelling, boggy feeling and arthrogram is used to confirm the diagnosis. Shoulder synovectomy includes subdeltoid bursa, subacromial bursa, synovectomy of all joint areas through arthrotomy by dividing the subscapularis near its insertion and anterior capsulotomy at its humeral attachment and excision of the synovial lining of the long head of biceps. Open synovectomy is performed through delto-pectoral interval. Synovectomy may be accomplished arthroscopically. Rotator cuff defects may be repaired.

Postoperatively arm is given rest in slight abduction by placing a pillow. Exercises are commenced 2–3 days after surgery. Early passive movements are given to control post-operative edema, pain and stiffness. Active exercises are delayed until healing of tendon repair is complete.

ARTHRODESIS

Arthrodesis is the surgical fusion of joint. With the advent of shoulder arthroplasty for destructive arthritis and injury and with the control of poliomyelitis and tuberculosis, there is very little indication for arthrodesis. Currently, the major indications for arthrodesis of glenohumeral joint include combined paralysis of deltoid and rotator cuff, uncontrolled instability. Glenohumeral arthrodesis eliminates all rotation and 120 degrees of the 180 degrees elevation of the shoulder. The most important function of the shoulder is to rotate the humerus so that the elbow flexion-extension positions the hand where it is needed. After fusion, no rotation and only 60 degrees of elevation of scapulothoracic joint is available, allowing the hand to reach below the hip pocket (Fig. 11.1) to the eyebrows (Fig. 11.2). The most critical position to consider in a fusion is the position of rotation. If the fusion is in more external rotation, the hand may reach to the top of the head but cannot reach the opposite axilla, belt buckle or the zipper. With the fusion in more internal

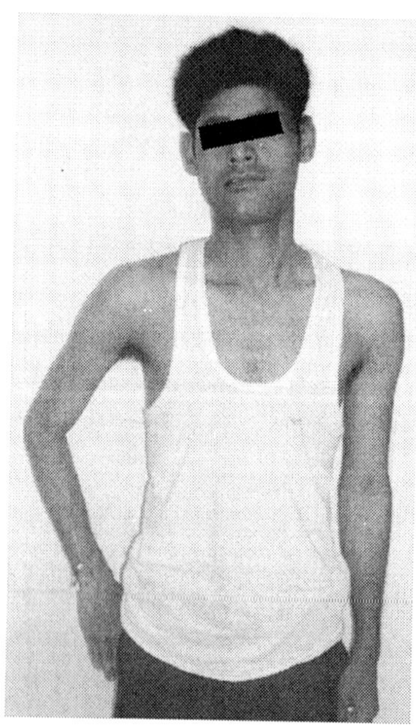

Fig. 11.1: Shoulder arthrodesis allowing hand to reach below the hip pocket

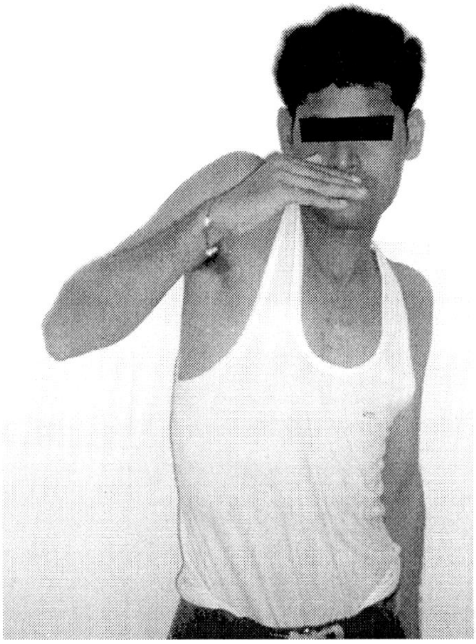

Fig. 11.2: Shoulder arthrodesis allowing the hand to reach eyebrows

rotation, the hand can reach the anal region but has difficulty in reaching the mouth. The position of elevation of the arm is less critical, but a fusion in excessive forward elevation or abduction causes a prominence of scapula and early fatigue of scapular muscles. A fusion in too much abduction also causes inability to lower the arm to the side of the body, creating inconvenience during ambulation and in recumbency. Rowe recommended fusion at 20° abduction, 30° of flexion and 40° of internal rotation; Hawkins and Neer recommended 25–40° abduction, 20–30° of flexion and 25–30° of internal rotation.

Indications of fusion include paralysis or destruction from trauma of both rotator cuff and deltoid muscles with functioning scapulothoracic muscles (trapezius, levator scapulae, rhomboids, pectoralis), above 6 years of age.

Contraindications of fusion include active infection, paralysis of both trapezius and serratus anterior muscles, instability, failed reconstructive procedure and contralateral fusion.

Intra-articular fusion is the simpler method, in which the joint is debrided and the articular cartilage, scar and dense subchondral bone are removed. Cancellous bone of the humeral head and glenoid is placed against each other with iliac crest bone graft, and the arm is fixed in the desired position by screws, wires or pins. Shoulder spica immobilization is applied for 3–6 months, until there is X-ray evidence of bone consolidation. Extra-articular technique is preferred in case of infection. Fusion is achieved by adding bone graft between the humeral head and the acromion or between the humeral neck and the medial aspect of scapula adjacent to the glenoid, avoiding the infective focus and fixed by internal fixator such as tension band wiring, plate and screw or narrow dynamic compression plate or external fixator. External fixator is preferred if the shoulder is infected. Intra-articular fusion can be combined with extra-articular fusion.

Preoperatively the patient must be told regarding the post-operative limitations. Postoperatively during the immobilization one should be encouraged to do active wrist and hand movements, static contraction of biceps and triceps. Following plaster removal measures for pain relief, elbow range of motion and strengthening, scapular muscles strengthening and functional re-education should be done.

Complications

Pseudoarthrosis, infection, reflex sympathetic osteodystrophy, fracture shaft of humerus, acromioclavicular arthritis and girdle pain.

BIBLIOGRAPHY

1. Charles A Rockwood, Fred Rick A. Matson, Michael A. Wirth: The shoulder (vol. II) 3rd edn. Saunders, 2005;655-781.
2. Charles S. Neer: Shoulder Reconstruction; WB Saunders, 1990; 143-269.
3. Katsuya Nobuhara: The shoulder - Its function and clinical aspects, 1st edn. World scientific Publishing Co. Ltd. 2003;472-92.
4. Lynn A Crosby: Total shoulder arthroplasty, American Academy of Orthopaedic Surgeons Jaypee Publ. 2004.
5. Richard J. Friedman: Total shoulder arthroplasty. The Orthopaedic Clinics of North America, 1998;377-565.

Index

Page numbers followed by *f* refer to figure.

T